Choriocarcinoma

UICC Monograph Series · Volume 3

Choriocarcinoma

Transactions of a Conference
of the International Union against Cancer

Edited by

James F. Holland · Myroslaw M. Hreshchyshyn

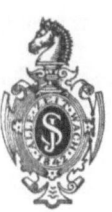

Springer-Verlag Berlin Heidelberg New York 1967

James F. Holland, M. D., Chief of Medicine A and Director, Cancer Clinical Research Center, Roswell Park Memorial Institute, Buffalo, N.Y.

Myroslaw M. Hreshchyshyn, M. D., Associate Professor of Obstetrics and Gynecology, State University of New York at Buffalo, N. Y., and Associate Cancer Research Gynecologist, Roswell Park Memorial Institute, Buffalo, N. Y.

ISBN 978-3-642-85909-0   ISBN 978-3-642-85907-6 (eBook)
DOI 10.1007/978-3-642-85907-6

Softcover reprint of the hardcover 1st edition 1967

Library of Congress Catalog Card Number 66-29099

Titel-Nr. 7515

Contents

Introduction (JAMES F. HOLLAND) 1

The Pathology of Trophoblastic Tumours, W. W. PARK* 3

Transplantation Immunity and the Trophoblast, R. E. BILLINGHAM* 9

Alternations of the Thymo-Lymphatic System in Malignant Trophoblastic Disease
J. H. NELSON* 18

Serial Passage of Choriocarcinoma of Women in The Hamster Cheek-Pouch, R. HERTZ* . 26

Synopsis of discussion I 32

Trophoblastic or Chorionic Tumors as Observed in the Philippines, H. ACOSTA-SISON* . . 33

The Natural History of Choriocarcinoma, D. P. C. CHAN* 37

Early Development of Choriocarcinoma, J. I. BREWER* and A. B. GERBIE 45

A Study of Choriocarcinoma. Its Incidence in India and Its Aetiopathogenesis, K. N. PAI* . 54

Observation on Some Aspects of Hydatidiform Mole and Choriocarcinoma in Indonesia,
A. SOEJOENOES, M. DJOJOPRANOTO*, and H. T. POEN 58

Synopsis of discussion II 59

The Mechanism of Action of Folic Acid Antagonists, J. F. HOLLAND* 60

Eight Years Experience with the Chemotherapy of Choriocarcinoma and Related Trophoblastic Tumors in Women, R. HERTZ* 66

On the Prevention and Treatment of Choriocarcinoma, C. P. MANAHAN*, R. ABAD, and
A. M. LOPEZ 72

Chemotherapeutic Prophylaxis Against the Development of Choriocarcinoma Following
the Removal of Hydatidiform Mole, K. KOGA* and K. MAEDA* 76

An Observation on the Prophylactic Use of Chemotherapy After Termination of Hydatidiform Mole, D. Chun*, T. Lu, and H. K. CHUNG 77

The Effect of Methotrexate in Trophoblastic Diseases, C. T. HSU*, T. F. WANG, S. E.
LIANG, H. P. HSU, W. T. TSAI, and S. Y. PEN 80

Methotrexate Treatment in Choriocarcinoma (Preliminary Report), K. L. LIEM* 81

Synopsis of discussion III 82

Urinary Excretion of Gonadotropin and the Estrogens in Hydatidiform Mole and Choriocarcinoma, B. ZONDEK and M. FINKELSTEIN* 84

Endocrinological Studies Relating to Trophoblastic Disease in Man, R. HERTZ* 94

Pelvic Angiography in the Management of Malignant Trophoblastic Disease, J. P. DE V.
HENDRICKSE*, W. P. COCKSHOTT, and D. M. JAMES 98

Diagnosis of Hydatidiform Mole and Related Trophoblastic Diseases. A Further Study of the Galli-Mainini Bioassay Test. KOESOEMOWARDOJO, I. W. GIRI, and M. DJOJOPRANOTO * 105

Comments on the Measurement of HCG as a Tumor Specific Substance, K. D. BAGSHAWE * 109

Urinary Estrogen Excretion in Chorionic Tumor Patients, K. KOGA * and K. MAEDA * . . 112

Quantitative Human Chorionic Gonadotropin Immunoassay, M. M. HRESHCHYSHYN * and N. R. ROSE 113

Synopsis of discussion IV 114

Chemotherapy of Chorionic Tumors, N. ISHIZUKA * 116

The Use of 6-Mercaptopurine with Methotrexate in the Treatment of Trophoblastic Tumors, K. D. BAGSHAWE * 119

Remissions Induced in Patients with Trophoblastic Tumors by 6-Diazo-5-Oxo-L-Norleucine (DON), D. A. KARNOFSKY *, R. B. GOLBEY, and M. C. LI * 126

Fundamental Problems of Chemotherapy of Choriocarcinoma, M. NATSUME * 135

Clinical Effects of Vinblastine in Chorionic Tumors, T. HASEGAWA *, G. OGAWA, T. KOBAYASHI *, M. NATSUME *, Y. ASHIDAKA, K. KOGA *, and G. NOZUE 136

The Clinical Evalution of Various Anticancer Agents on Chorionic Tumors, T. KOBAYASHI * 137

Chemotherapeutic and Immunological Considerations on the Response of Choriocarcinomas, M. C. LI * 138

Synopsis of discussion V 145

Integration of Treatment Methods in Trophoblastic Growths, M. M. HRESHCHYSHYN * and J. F. HOLLAND * 148

Synopsis of discussion VI 152

Appendix I 155

Appendix II 156

Appendix III 157

---

* = Attendance at meeting.

Participants

Conference on the Chemotherapy of Choriocarcinoma

Dr. H. Acosta-Sison, Professor of Obstetrics and Gynecology, University of Philippines, Manila, Philippines

Dr. Kenneth D. Bagshawe, Senior Lecturer in Medicine, Charing Cross Hospital Medical School, Fulham Hospital, London, England

Dr. Rupert Billingham, Professor of Medical Genetics, University of Pennsylvania, School of Medicine, Philadelphia 4, Pennsylvania, U.S.A.

Dr. Manuel Borja, Chief of Gynecology, University of Santo Thomas, Manila, Philippines

Dr. John Brewer, Professor of Obstetrics and Gynecology, Northwestern University, Chicago, Illinois, U.S.A.

Dr. Joseph H. Burchenal, Vice-President, Sloan-Kettering Institute for Cancer Research, New York, New York, U.S.A.

Dr. Donald P. C. Chan, Head, Department of Obstetrics and Gynaecology, University of Malaya, Kuala Lumpur, Malaysia

Dr. Daphne Chun, Professor of Obstetrics and Gynecology, University of Hong Kong, Hong Kong

Dr. Moeljono Djojopranoto, Chairman, Department of Pathology, School of Medicine, University of Airlangga, Surabaja, Indonesia

Dr. Michael Finkelstein, Associate Professor of Endocrinology, Hormone Research Laboratory, Hebrew University, Hadassah Medical School, Jerusalem, Israel

Dr. Toshio Hasegawa, Chairman, Chorionic Tumor Committee, Japanese Obstetrical and Gynecological Society, c/o Japanese Red Cross Central Hospital, Tokyo, Japan

Dr. Roy Hertz, Professor of Obstetrics and Gynecology, The George Washington University Medical School, Washington, D.C., U.S.A.

Dr. Paul Hendrickse, Associate Professor of Obstetrics and Gynecology, University of Ibadan, Ibadan, Nigeria

Dr. James F. Holland, Chief of Medicine A, Roswell Park Memorial Institute, Buffalo, New York 14203, U.S.A.

Dr. Myroslaw M. Hreshchyshyn, Associate Professor of Obstetrics and Gynecology, State University of New York at Buffalo, School of Medicine, Buffalo, New York 14214, U.S.A.

Dr. Chien-Tien Hsu, Dean, Taipei Medical College, P. O. Box Taipei No. 12110, Taipei, Taiwan, China

Dr. Naotaka Ishizuka, Professor of Obstetrics and Gynecology, Nagoya University School of Medicine, Nagoya, Japan

Dr. David A. Karnofsky, Member, Sloan-Kettering Institute for Cancer Research, New York, New York, U.S.A.

Dr. Takashi Kobayashi, Professor of Obstetrics and Gynecology, Tokyo University School of Medicine, Tokyo, Japan

Dr. Kohachiro Koga, Professor of Obstetrics and Gynecology, University of Kyushu School of Medicine, Fukuoka, Japan

Dr. Leopold G. Koss, Chief of Cytology, Sloan-Kettering Institute for Cancer Research, New York, New York, U.S.A.

Dr. Min C. Li, Director, Department of Medical Research, Nassau Hospital, Mineola, New York, U.S.A.

Dr. Khe Loen Liem, Department of Obstetrics and Gynecology, University of Indonesia, Djakarta, Indonesia

Dr. K. Maeda, Assistant Professor, Department of Obstetrics and Gynecology, Kuyshu University Hospital, Fukuoka, Japan

Dr. Constantino P. Manahan, Manila Doctors Hospital, Manila, Philippines

Dr. Misao Natsume, Professor of Obstetrics and Gynecology, Gifu Prefectural Medical College, Gifu, Japan

Dr. James H. Nelson, Associate Professor of Obstetrics and Gynecology, State University of New York, Downstate Medical Center, Brooklyn, New York, U.S.A.

Dr. W. Wallace Park, Department of Pathology, Queen's College, Dundee, Scotland

Dr. K. N. Pai, Professor of Medicine, Medical College, Trivandrum, Kerala, India

Dr. Basilio Valdes, Vice-President, Philippine Cancer Society, 310 San Rafael, P. O. Box 3066, Manila, Philippines

Introduction

The International Union Against Cancer convened a Conference on the Chemotherapy of Choriocarcinoma in Baguio City, Philippines to focus attention on the therapy of neoplasms of the trophoblast.

Cures of cancer are of concern to every man. The oldest therapy of cancer likely consisted of herbs, potions and incantations. Cures may first have been achieved in the murky annals of early civilization with local chemical cautery. The first successes of surgery are lost in antiquity and probably were amputations. Radiation therapy was first used for cure in the early years of the 20th century. Curability of the first cancer with drugs is a recent phenomenon: choriocarcinoma in 1956.

There are several known agencies of cure for choriocarcinoma and other trophoblastic neoplasia. Surgery, and now chemotherapy with methotrexate, actinomycin D, 6-mercaptopurine or vinblastine. As with other known curative methods for cancer, the distribution of talent and of resources remain the great task. Knowledge alone that cure exists is not enough. The worldwide distribution of skills should be easier with drugs for use in trophoblastic neoplasia, however, than the distribution of other curative approaches to other neoplasms has been.

The stated purposes of the Conference, thus, were to share information, experience and teaching so that no woman should die of choriocarcinoma in the farthest reaches of the world for lack of knowledge of what to do or how to do it; to identify the nature of, and reason for, the successful chemotherapeutic results in trophoblastic neoplasia (whether this be specificity of drugs, the nature of the allogenic graft or characteristics of the specific cells); and to determine the causes for failures (whether it be advanced and long-standing disease, inappropriate dosage regimens, or inherent resistance of the tumors treated). If this first chemotherapeutically curable cancer can serve as a model for the chemotherapy of other autochthonous tumors, the therapeutic principles may be useful for extrapolation to other tumors. Such unique characteristics as the technique of dosing and the drugs used, the biochemical parameters of diagnosis, the parasitic nature of the parent placenta from which the trophoblastic neoplasia arises, and immunologic considerations all were raised for consideration during the Conference.

The striking variation in incidence of trophoblastic neoplasia in different regions of the world implies that there are factors responsible which might be environmental and mutable, and offers a possibility of prevention. Since the effective chemotherapeutic regimens were developed in the Western world where the incidence of trophoblastic neoplasia is low, the Conference was deliberately held in the East where trophoblastic neoplasia is agonizingly common.

A new taxonomy was adopted at the Conference for clarity of international communication. This will be recommended to the UICC for adoption Appendix I. The Conference has borne fruit, in that an International Trophoblastic Neoplasia Study Group has been organized to test in prospect some of the questions raised at the Conference.

The Conference served as a suitable forum to recognize the significant and continuing contributions of Dr. ROY HERTZ to the chemotherapy of this group of neoplasms. A citation to Dr. HERTZ is reprinted in Appendix II, and his several cogent contributions are published in these transactions in the chronological order of their presentation.

The participants were indebted to Dr. MANUEL BORJA, the Chairman of the Local Arrangements Committee for outstanding performance, and so memorialized him. The Philippine Cancer Society graciously and effectively served as host.

Part of the expenses of the Conferences were generously supported by the Lederle Laboratories Division, American Cyanamid Co., the Upjohn Co., the Burroughs-Wellcome Co., Merck Sharpe & Dohme, Inc., and Hoffman-LaRoche, Inc.

James F. Holland, M. D.

The Pathology of Trophoblastic Tumours

W. WALLACE PARK

Department of Pathology, University of St. Andrews,
Queen's College, Dundee, Scotland

Gestational trophoblast has at least as wide a range of pathological behaviour as any other tissue, and a wider range than most. I believe that this requires emphasis for we are in some danger of holding too narrow a view of its pathological potential in general and its neoplastic potential in particular. At some stage in earliest development an important decision is made: some cells are destined to form the embryo, others to form trophoblast, and we have no reason to believe that the cells in the one group are any more or less prone to biological disturbance than those in the other. Certainly, the varied disturbances that we see in the foetus or new-born infant are more conspicuous than those which we see in trophoblast; but this is easily understandable. Tissue differentiation in the developing embryo is varied and complex; so also may be the expressions of damage. Trophoblast, on the other hand, is by comparison a simple tissue with little capacity for differentiation. It may indeed be affected by all the agents that can harm the embryo but a form of structure as limited as this cannot match in variability at least the *structural* expressions of disease that we see in the embryo. I have little doubt that many abortions are due to disorders of the trophoblast rather than of the embryo but we have not yet learned how to recognise them.

Our concern here is with trophoblastic neoplasia, and here there is ample variation. Exact comparison with neoplasms elsewhere is not possible because, for one thing, intra-uterine neoplasia of whatever kind, by its effects, demands treatment more urgently than neoplasia in other sites commonly does and so only rarely do we gain an inkling of what the natural history of the lesion would have been. Within this limitation, however, I believe that neoplastic trophoblast has as widely spread an intrinsic or biological potential as that of any other neoplastic tissue.

The essential morbid anatomical features of trophoblastic overgrowths are well known and I doubt whether the necropsy as such has much more information to provide. However, tissue obtained at necropsy as well as that obtained during life has undoubtedly more information to yield. Experimental observations are, and will continue to be, indispensable but we must always remember that observations made on the trophoblast of other animals may have but little relevance to trophoblast in the human. The "success story" of Methotrexate tells us that this is not always so but we should not too readily assume that further knowledge is likely to be gained only from the non-human experimental animal. The techniques of immunology, tissue culture,

1*

electron microscopy and cytogenetics, for example, have been applied but lightly as yet to the problems posed by the physiology and thus the pathology of human trophoblast.

I propose to describe some of the situations in which trophoblastic abnormality may cause diagnostic difficulty for the pathologist and, correspondingly, prognostic difficulty for the clinician, and in so doing shall refer to many if not most of the questions that remain so far from being answered.

The ordinary *placental polyp* should not cause diagnostic difficulty but it is a strange phenomenon and merits our thought. Here we have a fragment of virtually normal villous placenta that has remained in situ and achieved a peaceful symbiosis with the endometrium (histologically but not symptomatically) maintaining for itself a decidual microclimate. Such polyps are not common and are usually seen as a post-partum occurrence. Their trophoblast is thus aged, a fact that may explain the rarity with which they show trophoblastic hyperplasia.

So-called *benign chorionic invasion*, on the other hand, is well recognised as a not infrequent cause of diagnostic difficulty. Some degree of giant-cell permeation of the decidua is probably present at some stage of every pregnancy but its extent varies greatly. Some placental beds show no more than one giant-cell per sq. cm.; others show abundant cells that may be bizarre, histologically disturbing and not easy to distinguish from the cells of chorioncarcinoma. Most of these cells are almost certainly of trophoblastic origin but I myself have no doubt that from the other side, not only decidua but also myometrium may contribute multinucleated giant-cells to the population in the placental bed. Recently, LARSEN (1961) has gone so far as to say that in the rabbit at any rate foetal and maternal cells may

actually fuse, nuclei from both sources coming together to form symplastic masses. This is an intriguing interpretation of morphological appearances that has already stimulated fresh thought and new investigations. Whether this fusion occurs in the human, and, if so, what its physiological and pathological implications may be, remains to be determined. It is clearly of great potential relevance to the problems of graft-immunity posed by the foetal-maternal relationship, normal, or abnormal as in abortions and states of trophoblastic neoplasia.

Now let us turn to the mechanism of formation or mode of origin of the *hydatidiform mole*. I have already discussed this debatable matter elsewhere (PARK, 1959) and accordingly propose to do no more than mention briefly the main features of the differing views so as to place in perspective some relevant evidence derived from recent studies on sex chromatin and chromosomes in hydatidiform moles. According to one hypothesis (HERTIG and EDMONDS, 1940) primary death of the embryo in conjunction with continued secretory activity by the trophoblast results in (a) accumulation of fluid within the villus — since there is no embryonic circulation to carry it away, and (b) hyperplasia of the trophoblast in consequence of its being "stretched". According to another hypothesis which I have supported (PARK, 1959a) the primary disturbance lies in the trophoblast. This is, as we know, *structurally* abnormal, and it seems not unreasonable to postulate an associated *functional* abnormality of the trophoblast that brings about excessive absorption of fluid into the villi with consequent destruction of blood vessels, perhaps simply by pressure, and thus death of the embryo. The difference between the two hypotheses may be summarised thus: (a) embryonic death → fluid accumulation within villi → trophoblastic hyperplasia; (b) structural and functional abnormality of trophoblast → fluid accumulation within villi → embryonic death. Whether the trophoblastic abnormality is most properly to be regarded as hyperplasia, dysplasia or benign neoplasia is difficult to answer.

The chromosomal characteristics and distribution of sex chromatin within hydatidiform moles have been most recently reported by ATKIN at a Symposium in Dundee (1964). He (and his colleague Dr. KLINGER) found sex chromatin to be present in 47 of 53 hydatidiform moles; and, in 4 out of 6 that were cultured, there was a normal female chromosome complement. It may now be taken as a fact that the tissues of 80% or so of "ordinary" hydatidiform moles are chromatin-positive, and, with almost as much assurance, that most of these have a euploid XX chromosomal constitution. Hydatidiform moles may be accepted therefore to this extent as female conceptuses. Whatever the reason for this unusual sex incidence, and no adequate explanation has emerged so far, its occurrence virtually rules out simple embryonic death as the cause for the hydatidiform mole, for, if this were the whole explanation, moles should be, not predominantly chromatin-positive, but chromatin-positive and chromatin-negative in approximately equal number with a tendency towards chromatin-negative predominance in conformity with estimates of the primary sex ratio. Admittedly, the disproportion we see could be brought about by the operation of some hypothetical female-sex-linked lethal gene but this would not explain the great rarity of the male hydatidiform conceptus. It is difficult to accept that, of conceptuses dying during the first few weeks of pregnancy, only a minute proportion is male; indeed, as just mentioned, all the evidence points in the opposite direction. This is the main defect of the absent-embryonic-circulation hypothesis in this context: it fails in explanation of the negative instance. The hypothesis of primary trophoblastic abnormality, on the other hand, seems to me to be less vulnerable and better able to accomodate this new knowledge. The abnormality that is postulated, trophoblastic hyperplasia/dysplasia/neoplasia, may be a feature just of the "femaleness" of the conceptus. There is nothing scientifically improper in this suggestion. In the case of the thyroid, for example, we can do little more than ascribe the predominance of its hyperplasia/dysplasia/neoplasia in the female to just "femaleness". Further speculation in this matter is hardly warranted until we know much more of the chromosomal characteristics of trophoblast but I would just mention in conclusion the significant observation of MAKINO and his associates (1963) that hydatidiform moles, chorioadenomata destruentia and chorioncarcinomata show, in that order, increasing degrees of chromosomal aberrancy. The case for regarding trophoblastic abnormality as the main cause of hydatidiform molar development, and the hydrops and death of the embryo as secondary consequences, would appear to be gaining strength.

The trophoblastic overgrowth that characterises the hydatidiform mole is a common source of diagnostic difficulty. The question raised by each is: Will this lesion be followed by choriocarcinoma or not?, and we are as far from being able to give a certain answer as were our predecessors of last century. I suggested some time ago (PARK, 1959) that, rather than describe the varying degrees of molar trophoblastic hyperplasia in such terms as possibly, probably and certainly malignant, we should in practice report them as indicating a risk of subsequent choriocarcinoma of 1, 5 or 10%, and this procedure has been adopted in some places. Such a report is, of course, only one factor, though possibly the most important, to be considered in assessment of the individual patient: thus, the clinician might decide that hysterectomy is preferable to a 1 % risk of choriocarcinoma at age 40 but that even a 10 % risk is preferable to hysterectomy in a nulliparous patient aged 20. However, argument on how best to classify hydatidiform moles in terms of the risk they represent is already being rendered obsolete by the increasing use of chemotherapy. Indeed, I would go so far as to say that the combination of careful pregnancy-test supervision, a skilled clinician and chemotherapy has made the histological examination of a hydatidiform mole, for a short-term clinical purpose, virtually superfluous. Its importance for academic, and thus longterm clinical purposes remains as valid as ever.

The old belief is still justified that, in tissue which is or has been part of a hydatidiform mole, no matter how ominous the accompanying trophoblast may appear, the continued *presence of chorionic villi* favours a diagnosis of non-malignancy. Now this is a curious situation and merits study, and I consider that we would be wrong to continue passively to accept the association between persistence of villi and absence of choriocarcinoma, prognostically helpful though it be, as simply an empirical fact. It merits at least some analysis.

There are in fact some situations where the presence of villi amongst hyperplastic trophoblast is clearly *not* an absolute pointer to future behaviour. We assume, probably (but not necessarily) correctly, that the trophoblast which kills a patient by metastasis, say, 12 months after passage of a hydatidiform mole, has been derived from some part of the original covering trophoblast of that mole. Yet, when we had examined the mole a year

before death we saw hyperplastic trophoblast, and it was attached to villi. The obvious suggestion, that some focus of choriocarcinoma within the mole was 'missed' is scarcely acceptable any longer. As I have just stated, all attempts — and they have been many — to establish criteria for the certain recognition of the premalignant mole have so far failed. If there really were a discoverable, prognostically reliable lesion within such moles we would know of it by now. Such, at any rate, is my own view. At this early stage and in this context, therefore, the presence of villi is prognostically meaningless. It would thus appear that the relationship between trophoblast and villus in these circumstances is in some important way different from that obtaining in those *other* circumstances where the continuing presence of villi *is* of prognostically good significance. If we enquire further into the difference between these two sets of circumstances we find that the presence of villi is used as a criterion of prognostic significance almost always *in one situation only*, namely, in assessment of material obtained from the uterus 'abnormally long' after the passage of a hydatidiform mole. The term "abnormally long" cannot be defined with accuracy: suffice it to say that the problem is usually contained in material obtained one week or more after the mole has been passed, and these are the conditions in which, lacking a hysterectomy specimen, we diagnose chorioadenoma or mola destruens [invasive hydatidiform mole — Ed.]. It would appear that the trophoblast of a hydatidiform mole which behaves in this unusually tenacious or even penetrative way is at least no more, and may be intrinsically less, liable to malignant metastasis than that of the "ordinary", relatively non-invasive type of hydatidiform mole. The matter is not easy to establish with statistical certainty but it appears to be substantially true that this type of trophoblast, despite its much greater opportunity of access to vascular channels, is associated with subsequent choriocarcinoma no more frequently than is that of the non-invasive type of mole. It is therefore not the continued presence of villi as such that indicates a relatively good prognosis: rather it is that by them we recognise the lesion as a mola destruens, a lesion which we know from past experience to be much less dangerous than its trophoblast alone would suggest. The conclusion seems inescapable that we are dealing here with a type of trophoblast biologically quite different from that of the abovementioned hydatidiform mole that killed by choriocarcinomatous metastasis 12 months after its passage. The mola destruens is really a trophoblastic rodent ulcer. It has a variable growth rate, is locally destructive of tissue and has little tendency to metastasize as a choriocarcinoma.

We may carry analysis of the significance of persistent villi further. Some observers believe that chorionic mesoderm is formed by differentiation from trophoblast (HERTIG and ROCK, 1941), so there is at least a parallel possibility that villi found in the uterus in association with abnormal trophoblast, as in the mola destruens, are not always remnants of the original hydatidiform mole but new formations created by differentiation from the trophoblast and thus indicative of trophoblast of a certain biological type[1]. This concept has some relevance to one of the not infrequent peculiarities of choriocarcinoma, namely absence of a primary lesion in uterus or adnexa. Until the advent of chemotherapy, the uterus of a patient dead of metastatic choriocarcinoma was either absent (from hysterectomy) or virtually normal, and many indeed have been the uteri serially sectioned after death with negative results in patients

with multiple metastases. In most such patients the early history has been one of passage of a hydatidiform mole, no troublesome sequelae and, for a time, full clinical recovery. It seems likely that the trophoblast in these cases is metastasisingly malignant from an exceptionally early stage and is thus perhaps of *still another* biological type. The position may be (a) that abnormal trophoblast which, by differentiation, *can* form villi, has only a *locally* malignant potential: presence of villi and a relatively good prognosis therefore "go together", and (b) that abnormal trophoblast which *cannot*, by differentiation, form villi, has a *metastasisingly* malignant potential: absence of villi and a relatively poor prognosis therefore also "go together". This proposition does not have absolute validity. Thus, there is no evidence that the trophoblast which participates in "benign chorionic invasion" can form mesodermal villous tissue; also, I have seen a mass in the myometrium, present long enough to have formed for itself a virtual capsule and be mistaken at operation for a circumscribed myoma, yet histologically an undoubted villus-free choriocarcinoma and unaccompanied by metastases up to 3 years later. At the same time, it would be unwise to reject the possibility of the proposition's having at any rate some validity in application to frankly neoplastic trophoblast.

---

[1] This is also, incidentally, a possible explanation for the appearance of relatively large hydatidiform villi in such situations as the periphery of the lung (REED *et al.* 1959) where size of available blood vessels makes an embolic explanation difficult to accept. There are other possible explanations for this such as the existence of anastomotic channels (rather unlikely) or continued secretory activity by abnormal trophoblast in a villus that was normally-sized when it reached the lung, but the possibility of local differentiation of villous structure from trophoblast is at least admissible.

A closely related question is one first raised by ACOSTA-SISON (1955), whether the trophoblast of the conceptus may be carcinomatous from the first day of implantation, if not indeed from the day of its formation. There is no certain reason why this should not be possible. Reluctance to accept the possibility is based largely on a reluctance to believe that a carcinogenic stimulus can act so quickly. However, we have already to concede that in most cases of choriocarcinoma, where death may so rapidly follow the passage of a hydatidiform mole, the carcinogenic stimulus, whatever it be, has acted quite unusually swiftly. Furthermore, infants may be born with already far advanced somatic cancers such as neuro- and retino-blastoma or even disseminated cancer of uncertain origin, lesions which must certainly have started at a very early stage of development. The claim of DE RUYCK (1951) to have demonstrated a virus in hydatidiform mole and choriocarcinoma, which comes naturally to mind in this connection, remains tantalisingly unconfirmed. Progress in virological technique during the years since then undoubtedly warrants some further search.

I have commented on only some of the many unusual features of trophoblastic neoplasia, and I have done so intentionally in a largely speculative way. My reason for this is a belief that we have, over the past decade, reached a stage in our knowledge of trophoblastic neoplasia where increased understanding is more likely to be gained by the closer application of the newer techniques of investigation than by wider application of the old techniques; and that, with the change in emphasis from, for example, light microscopy to electron microscopy, and from mitotic appearances to cytogenetics, speculation and hypothesis are both acceptable and respectable. The need for new knowledge has been made all the greater and more urgent by the very success of chemotherapy for it appears as though much of the material we require for the purpose will disappear, fortunately and unfortunately, with the disappearance of the patient dead of chorioncarcinoma.

References

ACOSTA-SISON, H., Can the implanting trophoblasts of the fertilized ovum develop immediately into chorionepithelioma? *Amer. J. Obstet. Gynec.* 69, 442—446 (1955).

ATKIN, N. B., Sex chromatin and chromosome studies in trophoblast. In: *Proc. of Symposium on the Early Conceptus*, ed. PARK, W. W., pp. 130—134. Dundee: D. C. Thomson, 1965.

HERTIG, A. T., and EDMONDS, H. W., Genesis of hydatidiform mole. *Arch. Path.* 30, 260—291 (1940).

—, and ROCK, J., Two human ova of the previllous stage, having an ovulation age of about eleven and twelve days respectively. *Contr. Embryol. Carneg. Instn.* 29, 127—126 (1941).

LARSEN, J. F., Electron microscopy of the implantation site in the rabbit. *Amer. J. Anat.* 109, 319—325 (1961).

MAKINO, S., SASAKI, M. S., and FUKUSCHIMA, T., Preliminary notes on the chromosomes of human chorionic lesions. *Proc. Japan Acad.*, 39, 54 (1963).

PARK, W. W., Disorders arising from the human trophoblast. *In: Modern Trends in Pathology*, ed. COLLINS, D. H., pp. 180—211. London: *Butterworth*, 1959.

— Aspects of choriocarcinoma in the female. *Ann. N. Y. Acad. Sci.* 80, 152—160 (1959a).

REED, S., COE, J. I., and BERGQUIST, J., Invasive hydatidiform mole metastatic to the lungs. Report of a case. *Obstet. and Gynec.* 13, 749—753 (1959).

RUYCK, R. DE, Mise en evidence du virus choriotrope dans quatre cas de mole hydatiforme, et dans un cas de metastase pulmonaire de chorio-epitheliome. *Bull. Ass. franç.* 38, 252—268 (1951).

Transplantation Immunity and the Trophoblast

R. E. BILLINGHAM

*Department of Medical Genetics, University of Pennsylvania School of Medicine
Philadelphia, Pa.*

1. Introduction: Principles of transplantation immunology

Transplantation immunology is concerned with the genetically determined incompatibilities consistently displayed when grafts of cells, tissues or organs are exchanged between members of an outbred population. The cellular isoantigens responsible for inciting a host to respond against a homograft — the *homograft reaction* — are usually referred to as *transplantation antigens*. These antigens are determined by co-dominant *histocompatibility genes* and vary considerably in their relative strengths or sensitizing potencies. There is no evidence of any tissue specificity in transplantation immunology: the full complement of antigens determined by an animal's histocompatibility genes seems to be expressed by all the living, nucleate cells in its body, though cells of different types may differ quantitatively with respect to their content of these antigens.

Although the serologically detectable isoantigenic specificities of the erythrocytes of rodents include some that are determined by important histocompatibility genes, there is no evidence that these cells can elicit sensitivity to homografts of normal tissues. They may be ineffective vehicles for the transportation of antigens to immunologically reactive sites, or their specificities may be inadequately represented or inappropriately located.

At present our knowledge of the intracellular location and biochemical nature of the substances responsible for provoking homograft sensitization is rudimentary and derives almost exclusively from studies on lymphoid tissues and tumors of mice and rats. The antigenic specificities concerned appear to be closely associated with lipoprotein components of intracellular membranes and certainly they are on cell surfaces too.

There is a wealth of evidence that the principal seats of response to solid tissue homografts are the regional or draining lymph nodes. Most authorities believe that the reaction provoked by homografts of skin and other solid tissues that establish vascular and lymphatic connections with their hosts is closely related to drug and bacterial allergies and experimental autoimmune diseases. The common feature of these various sensitivities is that they all seem to be put into effect by blood-borne, immunologically activated cells of the lymphocytic series, in contradistinction to humoral antibodies. One of the most consistent and striking histological features of the process of homograft destruction is that it is preceded and accompanied by the infiltration of mononuclear cells. Various lines of evidence indicate that some kind of *local* engagement or interaction of these adventitious cells with antigenic matter in the graft culminates in its destruction, though the details of the process are still open to conjecture.

This classical cellular response to homografts is usually, though not necessarily, accompanied by a humoral one, though there is little evidence that the antibodies, identifiable *in vitro* as haemagglutinins, haemolysins, leucoagglutinins, cytotoxins, etc. play any significant role in the destruction of solid tissue homografts. Most authorities believe that the antigenic determinants corresponding to some histocompatibility genes can in some way provoke both humoral and cellular responses.

Detailed treatments of the various topics discussed above, and relevant bibliographies, will be found in reviews by BILLINGHAM and SILVERS (1963; 1965) and by RUSSELL and MONACO (1964).

2. Special sites and tissues

A few privileged or favored sites in the body are known in which small implants of tissue of alien origin may acquire a blood supply and yet enjoy prolonged, if not indefinite, acceptance by the host. Familiar examples include the brain, the anterior chamber of the eye, and the cheek pouch of the Syrian hamster (BILLINGHAM and SILVERS, 1962; RUSSELL and MONACO, 1964). The uniqueness of each of these sites seems to depend upon an incompleteness of the physiological pathways necessary for the evocation of a state of sensitivity — i. e., there is a break in the afferent pathway of the immunological reflex. The privileged status of both the brain and the hamster's cheek pouch seems to be a consequence of the absence of regional lym-

phatic drainage systems, so that there is no pathway to transmit an antigenic stimulus to a seat of response. However, in both sites an existing state of sensitivity is fully effective since blood vessels, bearing immunologically activated lymphocytic cells, constitute the efferent pathway of the immunological reflex.

Cartilage is almost unique in that it is an immunologically privileged *tissue*, capable of surviving transplantation even into a specifically sensitized host. Lack of blood vessels in such grafts and distinctive physico-chemical properties of the ground substance of this tissue are believed to be responsible for the complete invulnerability of the chondrocytes to transplantation immunity (BILLINGHAM and SILVERS, 1962).

3. The mammalian fetus as a homograft

Every pregnancy in an outbred mammalian population represents an intimate, natural parabiotic union and consequent exposure of the mother to fetal tissue she is potentially capable of reacting against immunologically. This follows from the fact that the fetus inherits from its father a variable number of transplantation antigens that are foreign to (i. e., not represented in) the mother. With the exception of parthenogenesis, the only situation where a fetus cannot confront its mother with any foreign antigens is where both its mother and its father are members of the same isogenic strain.

Consequently, ever since the basic principles of transplantation immunology first became established, biologists have sought to explain why, unlike homografts transplanted to nearly every site in the body, naturally implanted embryos in the uterus normally fail to provoke effective sensitization on the part of the mother. In all natural pregnancies the magnitude of the immunogenetic disparity between fetus and mother is necessarily restricted by the fact that the former inherits half its complement of histocompatibility genes from the latter. However, a difference with respect to only one or two major histocompatibility genes is all that is required to provoke reactions of maximal intensity (BILLINGHAM and SILVERS, 1963). Nevertheless, it is worth mentioning that what must represent much greater degrees of histoincompatibility have been achieved experimentally by transfer of fertilized eggs resulting from a mating between one pair of individuals to the uterus of a genetically unrelated third party — i. e., an experimental foster mother. Such experimental foster pregnancies still seem to defy the "laws of transplantation" by proceeding to term with no overt immunological complications (BILLINGHAM, 1964). Successful transfers of zygotes have been reported in mice, rats, rabbits, sheep and cattle.

Even more impressive is the consistent failure of all attempts to prejudice the incidence or course of *heterospecific* pregnancies — i. e., those resulting from matings between genetically dissimilar parents — by sensitization of the mother with homografts of the father's skin. LANMAN, DINERSTEIN and FIKRIG (1962) failed to compromise the success of foster pregnancies in rabbits by grafting the intended foster mother with skin from both parents of the subsequently transferred blastocysts.

Numerous hypotheses have been advanced to account for the success of the fetus as a homograft in either normal or specifically presensitized mothers (BILLINGHAM, 1964). The three most important of these explanations are enunciated below and considered in relation to the evidence bearing upon them.

a) The fetus is antigenically immature.
The very plausible idea that mothers

tolerate the growth of their embryos since the latter don't develop their isoantigenic individuality until late in ontogeny was put forward by LITTLE in 1924. However, so far as the fetus *per se* is concerned, this hypothesis was decisively refuted when evidence was forthcoming that transplantation antigens appear very early in embryonic life. They are demonstrable in the chick embryo by the fourth day of incubation, and in mouse embryos sooner than the 12th day of gestation (BILLINGHAM, 1964; BILLINGHAM and SILVERS, 1963).

Tests conducted in mice have shown that paternally inherited transplantation antigens are present in the placenta too (BILLINGHAM, 1964). For example, it has been shown that if placental tissue grafts from F_1 hybrid mouse embryos are implanted into specifically presensitized hosts of the maternal strain (i. e., hosts which have been inoculated with cells of the paternal strain) they are destroyed in a peremptory manner (SIMMONS and RUSSELL, 1962). This establishes the susceptibility of at least one component of this composite organ to transplantation immunity.

b) The uterus is an immunologically privileged site. Several limes of indirect evidence make it appear unlikely that any kind of privileged status of the uterine environment underlies the exemption of the fetus from the usual fate of homografts. In man, *non-uterine* tissues, such as the pelvic ileum or rectum, the fallopian tubes or the peritoneum may form implantation sites for fertilized eggs and subsequent attachment sites for the placentas. Despite these heterotopic attachments, it is well-established that ectopic pregnancies may proceed more or less normally for considerable periods and, occasionally, even to term (JARCHO, 1949; THIERSCH, 1941; WEINER, 1944). When fetal death does occur under these condititons, homograft reactivity on the part of the mother has never been invoked to account for it.

Naturally occurring ectopic pregnancies in animals are rare. However, in rodents segmenting eggs that have been caused to become attached to the mesenteries, or have been transferred beneath the renal capsules of histoincompatible hosts, still develop into normal embryos (Billingham, 1964).

Compelling evidence that the uterus has no distinctive properties that make it a favorable site for implantation of antigenically foreign embryos derives from Schlesinger's (1962) careful studies on tumor grafts implanted into the uterine horns of mice and rats. Only when tumors and their hosts were of the same immunogenetic constitution did the grafts grow successfully. Tumor homografts survived only for a short time in normal hosts and were rejected in accelerated fashion if implanted into presensitized animals, irrespective of whether the latter were non-pregnant, pseudo-pregnant or pregnant in one uterine horn.

A possible criticism of this experimental design is that the tumor homografts may have outgrown the uterine lining, so that their destruction was actually brought about as a result of their penetration of *extra-uterine* tissue. That this is not the case has been shown by Poppa *et al.* (1964) using test homografts of a normal, non-invasive tissue — parathyroid gland — implanted into the uterus of rats. Evidently then, transplantation immunity can both be evoked and expressed in the uterine milieu in a perfectly typical manner.

All the evidence reviewed so far sustains the view that whatever it is that prevents a fetus from sensitizing its mother, or renders it invulnerable to an extant state of sensitivity, must be associated with components of the fetus itself.

c) There is a physiological barrier between mother and fetus. As already mentioned, one of the most striking immunological properties of the fetus is its normal, virtually complete resistance to a state of sensitivity specifically directed against its own paternally inherited transplantation antigens. (However, we must not overlook the possible significance of suggestive evidence that habitual spontaneous abortion in women may be associated with a heightened degree of sensitivity to their husbands' transplantation antigens) (Bardawil *et al.*, 1962). In those species with placentas in which maternal blood is actually in contact with the fetal trophoblast — eg., man and rabbit — this resistance expresses itself in its most dramatic form, since here we have foreign cells of fetal origin chronically exposed to the cellular vehicles of homograft immunity — i. e., activated cells of the lymphocytic series.

Only one hypothesis can account for these facts: mother and fetus are completely separated by an anatomical barrier that not only prevents sensitization of the mother in respect of fetal transplantation antigens, but fully protects the fetus from an experimentally evoked state of specific sensitivity directed against it. There has long been agreement that the principal protective factor is the complete separation of the maternal and fetal blood circulations. However, this explanation is insufficient in that it does not take into account the large area over which living fetal and maternal tissues are so intimately juxtaposed. As one might anticipate, increasing attention became focused upon the fetal trophoblast since this represents an unbroken frontier component.

The idea that the placenta could function as a barrier if its trophoblast cells were non-antigenic was put forward many years ago by Witebsky and his associates

(OETTINGEN and WITEBSKY, 1928; WI-TEBSKY and REICH, 1932) on the basis of their observation that human placental villi are deficient in blood group antigens.

Almost decisive evidence that it is indeed the trophoblast that constitutes the immunologically protective barrier or buffer zone between mother and fetus has been presented by SIMMONS and RUSSELL (1962). These investigators have analyzed the histocompatibility characteristics of mouse placental tissue at various stages of its development. They studied grafts from F_1 hybrid embryos transplanted to adult hosts of the maternal strain since, under these conditions, the accidental inclusion of maternal cells in fetal tissue grafts cannot influence the host immunologically.

Seven-day-old mouse conceptuses were separated into their trophoblastic and embryonic portions and implanted beneath the renal capsules of specifically sensitized maternal strain hosts. The embryonic grafts underwent prompt destruction, but those of trophoblastic tissue displayed marked proliferative activity on the part of the giant cells with the formation of typical blood spaces. These grafts survived just as well and as long as if they had been transplanted to genetically compatible hosts.

Additional evidence that the mouse's trophoblast is an ineffective source of transplantation antigens was obtained from studies on fertilized ova or blastocysts transplanted heterotopically beneath the renal capsule or to the spleen (KIRBY, 1963; SIMMONS and RUSSELL, 1962). In genetically compatible hosts such grafts develop into "tumors" of trophoblast giant cells with a life-span of about two weeks. When F_1 hybrid ova were transplanted to normal maternal strain hosts their life-span gave no evidence of curtailment, nor did they elicit a detectable level of sensitivity in their hosts. Furthermore, there was no cellular response to such grafts even when they were implanted into specifically presensitized animals. Only when ova produced by mating parents of one isogenic strain were implanted beneath the renal capsules of specifically *hyperimmunized* mice of a third strain, manifesting high titers of *circulating* haemagglutinins, did the grafts fail to proliferate (SIMMONS, 1963).

The results of SCHLESINGER's (1964) recent studies on the absorption of isohaemagglutinins in mouse embryonic and trophoblastic tissue are also consonant with these findings. He found that whereas the whole placentas of embryos from upwards of $10\frac{1}{2}$ days show a constant and relatively high level of antigenic activity, trophoblastic growths resulting from grafts of $2\frac{1}{2}$—$3\frac{1}{2}$ day old fertilized eggs in the crytorchid testes of adult homologous hosts were without demonstrable serological activity.

There is also evidence that the trophoblast is sometimes capable of exerting its immunological protective role even where *species specific* antigenic differences are involved. This follows from the fact that healthy interspecific hybrid offspring may be born following matings between horses and donkeys; zebras and donkeys; cattle, bison and yak in different combinations; etc. (GRAY, 1954). KIRBY's (1962) demonstration that mouse blastocysts transplanted to *rat* kidneys produce flourishing trophoblast which invades and phagocytoses the surrounding tissue, closely resembling its behavior in a host of its *own* species, whereas a mouse embryo divested of its trophoblast provokes a massive cellular response, is in accord with this thesis.

All the available experimental evidence suggests that normal trophoblast cells fail to elaborate or express *transplantation* antigens in an immunologically effective manner. In this respect they bear at least a superficial resemblance to mammalian erythrocytes. KIRBY and his associates (1964) have recently obtained evidence that hints at the basis of this immunological "inertness" of the trophoblast. Electron microscopy reveals that *every* trophoblast cell is surrounded by an amorphous shell of fibrinoid material and that the thickness of this shell is related to the degree of genetic disparity between the mother and her conceptus. Hence the immunological quarantining of the trophoblast may bear some resemblance to that of cartilage in the manner in which it is brought about.

The results of a recent small-scale investigation of the fate of homografts of normal trophoblast, obtained from 2—3 month therapeutic abortions, to patients with inoperable carcinoma of the cervix are difficult to interpret (LAJOS et al. 1964). Evidence is presented that under conditions of hyperestrogenism the villous stroma degenerates whereas the trophoblast proliferates. In the absence of intensive estrogen therapy of the host, however, such grafts succumb to a homograft reaction within five weeks.

4. Chorionepitheliomas

The failure of normal trophoblast to express transplantation antigens in an immunologically effective form is consistent with the distinctive immunological properties of its malignant derivatives — choriocarcinomas — in man. It is now generally recognized that most of these highly invasive tumors originate from the chorionic epithelium of the fetus and develop in the mother within a highly variable interval after termination of the offending gestation. The successful growth and metastatic dissemination of these tumors is remarkable in view of their *fetal* origin — i. e., they are homografts.

Cognizance of the immunogenetically alien nature of these tumors has prompted attempts to arrest their growth immunologically (CINADER et al., 1961; DAUSSET, 1962; DONIACH et al., 1958; HACKETT and BEECH, 1961; MATHÉ et al., 1964; ROBINSON et al., 1963). These simply entail repeated intradermal injection of patients with leucocyte concentrates and/or skin grafts from their husbands. Unfortunately, these have been uniformly unsuccessful; a finding which is completely consistent with the distinctive properties of normal trophoblast. Of possible relevance here is the well-established empirical fact that homografts of many tumors in rodents are capable of over-riding degrees of histoincompatibility that would procure destruction of homografts of skin and other normal tissues. Also pertinent to the behavior of choriocarcinomas, in view of the fact that they secrete gonadotropins, is the fact that homografts of endocrine tissues are, under certain circumstances, less susceptible to transplantation immunity than grafts of non-endocrine tissues when only minor histocompatibility differences are involved (RUSSELL and MONACO, 1964).

Several reports have appeared that women with choriocarcinomas may display an *impaired* capacity to reject grafts of their husbands' skin, yet reject grafts from unrelated donors with normal vigor (MATHÉ et al., 1964; ROBINSON et al., 1963).

So far as I am aware the mononuclear cell infiltration which is almost invariably associated with homograft reactivity has never been observed in deposits of these tumors, either in untreated subjects or in those who have received homografts of their husband's skin. It is interesting to recall that, from a study of these tumors, HACKETT and BEECH (1961) concluded that choriocarcinomas are effectively non-antigenic. "... exhibiting the same mechanism or properties of physiologic non-antigenicity (whatever they may be) that exist in normal placenta".

Certain properties of these tumors hint that they are not always completely devoid of isoantigenic activity. Their spontaneous regression rate is relatively high, and a high proportion of apparently complete remissions of the disease can be obtained by treatment of female patients with amethopterin and other chemotherapeutic agents which might conceivably act in conjunction with a weak immune response on the part of the patient (HERTZ et al., 1961). However, if isoimmunization does contribute to these remissions, it does not seem to be accompanied by the appearance of humoral antibodies capable of reacting with the husband's red cell antigens (SCHMIDT and HERTZ, 1961). The ineffectiveness of chemotherapy in male patients with choriocarcinoma where there is, of course, complete genetic compatibility, is to some extent consistent with the view that in females isoimmunization and chemotherapy may act synergistically to check the growth of these tumors (LI et al., 1958).

Finally, since chemotherapy seems to be more effective if initiated soon after the onset of the disease, it is worth considering whether some of these tumors are feebly antigenic and that they induce some degree of *immunological tolerance* in the patient in respect of paternally inherited antigens. If this does happen, then the response of such a tolerant patient to chemotherapy would be little better than that of a genetically tolerant male subject. Indeed, the observed specifically diminished reactivity of some patients to grafts of their husbands' skin (MATHÉ et al., 1964; Robinson et al., 1963) hints that they may have been rendered partially

tolerant. The principle that tolerance of tissue homografts may sometimes be induced through exposure of *adult animals* to solid tissue homografts in certain sites is well-established on an empirical basis (BILLINGHAM and SILVERS, 1964). Most of the examples relate to situations where relatively minor histoincompatibilities are involved and the grafts are of endocrine origin (BILLINGHAM and SILVERS, 1965).

5. Conclusions

It is an unfortunate fact that our knowledge of the biology of choriocarcinomas is severely handicapped by the fact that these tumors are either extremely rare, or perhaps never occur, in laboratory mammals (SLYE et al., 1924; WILLIS, 1948). Various lines of evidence have been reviewed which suggest that, unlike homografts of other types of tumor in man, implants of choriocarcinomatous tissue into normal individuals should usually grow indefinitely, with only occasional spontaneous regressions. If animal experimentation were possible, then elucidation of the nature of the spontaneous regressions could easily be elucidated.

When appropriate techniques for typing, extracting and assaying transplantation antigens in man become available it will obviously be possible to determine the basis of the non- or only very feeble antigenicity of normal trophoblastic cells and their malignant variants. However, it seems unlikely that this will open up any hope of an immunological therapy based on transplantation isoantigens. Nevertheless, evidence that *organ specific* antigens are probably associated with trophoblast (HULKA and BRINTON, 1963; STEBLAY, 1962) indicates that we cannot entirely exclude the possibility of devising an immunotherapy.

References

BARDAWIL, W. A., MITCHELL, G. W., McKEOGH, R. P., and MARCHANT, D. J., Behaviour of skin homografts in human pregnancy. *Amer. J. Obstet. Gynec.* 84, 1283—1295 (1962).

Billingham, R. E., Transplantation immunity and the maternal-fetal relation. *New Engl. J. Med.* 270, 667—672, 720—725 (1964).

—, and Silvers, W. K., Studies on cheek pouch skin homografts in the Syrian hamster. In: *Transplantation*, Ciba Foundation Symposium, eds. G. E. W. Wolstenholme, and Cameron, M. P., p. 90. Boston: Little, Brown, 1962.

— —, Sensitivity to homografts of normal tissues and cells. *Ann. Rev. Microbiol.* 17, 531—564 (1963).

— —, Immunological aspects of tissue transplantation. In: *Immunological Diseases*, ed. M. Samter, p. 172. Boston: Little, Brown, 1965.

— —, Studies on homografts of fetal and infant skin and further observations on the anomalous properties of pouch skin grafts in hamsters. *Proc. roy. Soc. B* 161, 168—190 (1964).

Cinader, B., Hayley, M. A., Rider, W. D., and Warwick, O. H., Immunotherapy of patient with choriocarcinoma. *Can. med. Ass. J.* 84, 306—309 (1961).

Dausset, J., Leucocytes, platelets and human homografts. *Vox Sang. (Basel)* 7, 257—266 (1962).

Doniach, I., Crookston, J. H., and Cope, T. I., Attempted treatment of patient with choriocarcinoma by immunization with her husband's cells. *J. Obstet. Gynec. Brit. Empire.* 65, 553—556 (1958).

Gray, A. P., Mammalian hybrids: a check list with bibliography. (Technicial Communication No. 10.) Prepared by Commonwealth Bureau of Animal Breeding and Genetics, Edinburgh, Scotland 1954.

Hackett, E., and Beech, M., Immunological treatment of case of choriocarcinoma. *Brit. med. J.*, 1961 II, 1123—1126.

Hertz, R., Lewis, J., and Lipsett, M. B., Five years' experience with the chemotherapy of metastatic choriocarcinoma and related trophoblastic tumors in women. *Amer. J. Obstet Gynec.* 82, 631—640 (1961).

Hulka, J. F., and Brinton, V., Antibody to trophoblast during early postpartum period in toxemic pregnancies. *Amer. J. Obstet. Gynec.* 86, 130—134 (1963).

Jarcho, J., Ectopic pregnancy, with special reference to abdominal pregnancy. *Amer. J. Surg.* 77, 273—313 and 423—455 (1949).

Kirby, D. R. S., Reciprocal transplantation of blastocysts between rats and mice. *Nature (Lond.)* 194, 785—786 (1962).

Kirby, D. R. S., Development of mouse blastocyst transplanted to the spleen. *J. Reprod. Fertil.* 5, 1—12 (1963).

—, Billington, W. D., Bradbury, S., and Goldstein, D. J., Antigen barrier of the mouse placenta. *Nature (Lond.)* 204, 548—549 (1964).

Lajos, L., Görcs, J., Szekely, J., Csaba, I., and Domany, S., The immunologic and endocrinologic basis of successful transplantation of human trophoblast. *Amer J. Obstet. Gynec.* 89, 595—605 (1964).

Lanman, J. T., Dinerstein, J., and Fikrig, S., Homograft immunity in pregnancy: lack of harm to fetus from sensitization of mother. *Ann. N.Y. Acad. Sci.* 99, 706—716 (1962).

Li, M. C., Hertz, R., and Bergenstal, D. M., Therapy of choriocarcinoma and related trophoblastic tumors with folic acid and purine antagonists. *New Eng. J. Med.* 259, 66—74 (1958).

Little, C. C., Genetics of tissue transplantation in manmals. *J. Cancer Res.* 8, 75—95 (1924).

Mathé, G., Dausset, J., Heruet, E., Amiel, J. L., Colombani, J., and Brule, G., Immunological studies in patients with placental choriocarcinoma. *J. nat. Cancer Inst.* 33, 193—208 (1964).

Oettingen, Kj. V., u. Witebsky, E., Plazenta und Blutgruppe. *München med. Wschr.* 75, 385—386 (1928).

Poppa, G., Simmons, R. L., David, D. S., and Russell, P. S., The uterus as a recipient site for parathyroid homotransplantation. *Transplantation* 2, 496—502 (1964).

Robinson, E., Shulman, J., Ben-Hur, N., Zuckerman, H., and Neuman, Z., Immunological studies and behaviour of husband and foreign homografts in patients with chorionepithelioma. *Lancet*, 1963 I, 300—302.

Russell, P. S., and Monaco, A. P., *The biology of tissue transplantation*. Boston: Little, Brown, 1964.

Schlesinger, M., Uterus of rodents as site for manifestation of transplantation immunity against transplantable tumors. *J. nat. Cancer Inst.* 28, 927—945 (1962).

—, Serologic studies of embryonic and trophoblastic tissues of the mouse. *J. Immunol.* 93, 255—263 (1964).

Schmidt, P. J., and Hertz, R., Blood group factors in women with choriocarcinoma as compared with those of their husbands. *Amer. J. Obstet. Gynec.* **82**, 651—653 (1961).

SIMMONS, R. L., and RUSSELL, P. S., Antigenicity of mouse trophoblast. *Ann. N. Y. Acad. Sci.* **99**, 717—732 (1962).

—, Potential immunologic interactions at the placental site. In: *Transcript of the Second Rochester Trophoblast Conference*, ed. H. A. THIEDE, p. 389—402 (1963).

SLYE, M., HOLMES, H. F., and WELLS, H. G., Primary spontaneous tumors of the uterus in mice with review of comparative pathology of uterine neoplasms: studies on incidence and inheritability of spontaneous tumors in mice. *J. Cancer Res.* **8**, 96—118 (1924).

STEBLAY, R. W., Localization in human kidney of antibodies formed in sheep against human placenta. *J. Immunol.* **88**, 434—442 (1962).

THIERSCH, J. B., Intra-abdominal pregnancy. *Med. J. Aust.* **2**, 127 (1941).

THOMAS, R. C., Primary abdominal and primary ovarian pregnancy, with report of one case of each variety. *J. Obstet. Gynec. Brit. Emp.* **50**, 189—195 (1943).

WEINER, J. J., Primary abdominal pregnancy: a case report. *Amer. J. Surg.* **65**, 288—289 (1944).

WILLIAMS, C., A case of primary peritoneal pregnancy. *Med. J. Aust.* **2**, 326 (1941).

WILLIS, R. A., *Pathology of Tumors*. London: Butterworth 1948.

WITEBSKY, E., u. REICH, H., Zur Gruppenspezifischen Differenzierung der Placentaorgane. *Klin. Wschr. II*, 1960—1961 (1932).

Alternations of the Thymo-Lymphatic System in Malignant Trophoblastic Disease

JAMES H. NELSON, JR., M. D.

Department of Obstetrics and Gynecology State University of New York, Downstate Medical Center Brooklyn, New York, Visiting Investigator, Division of Clinical Chemotherapy Sloan-Kettering Institute of Cancer Research, and the Department of Medicine, Cornell University Medical College New York, New York

Aided by grant No. T—328 A from the American Cancer Society

The absolute lymphocyte count bears a relation to chorionic gonadotropin in patients with malignant trophoblastic tumors. Certain changes are known to occur in lymphoid tissue in normal pregnancy and in malignant trophoblastic tumors. 1. It has been shown by numerous investigators (JOLLY and LIEURE, 1930; PERSIKE, 1940), that the thymus atrophies during pregnancy and regenerates in the puerperium in small animals. 2. It has also been shown that estrogen and cortisone produce a reversible atrophy of the thymus (DOUGHERTY and WHITE, 1945; PLAGGE, 1941). 3. Atrophy of the thymus leads to a secondary regression in the size and activity of the remainder of lymphoid tissue in the body (METCALF, 1960). 4. Cortisol also acts directly on lymph nodes to produce a diminution of size of the nodes and depletion of small lymphocytes as well (DOUGHERTY and WHITE, 1945).

We know very little of the thymus in normal pregnancy in humans. HAMMAR (1926) has, however, reported on 2 accidental deaths in pregnancy which showed thymic atrophy.

A number of investigators have shown that total circulating lymphocytes or absolute lymphocyte counts are decreased in women during normal pregnancy. Perhaps the most comprehensive study is that by RATH, et al., (1950). We have shown absence of germinal centers in lymph nodes during normal pregnancy (NELSON and HALL, 1964). This change has been shown to last for 4—6 weeks in the puerperium (NELSON and HALL, 1965) (Fig. 1 and 2). If we accept germinal centers as sites of lymphocyte production, then the lymphopenia in pregnancy is understandable. Apparently these changes are secondary to the increased estrogen and cortisol levels in pregnancy. Whether the thymus atrophies in pregnancy and contributes to the picture is not known. DAMESHEK, et al. have recently shown lymphopenia in those adults with thymectomy or radiation to the thymus suggesting that the system works the same in humans (ADNER et al., 1964).

Changes in choriocarcinoma

A. Lymph nodes

I have been able to study the lymph nodes of only 2 patients with malignant trophoblastic tumors. They demonstrate

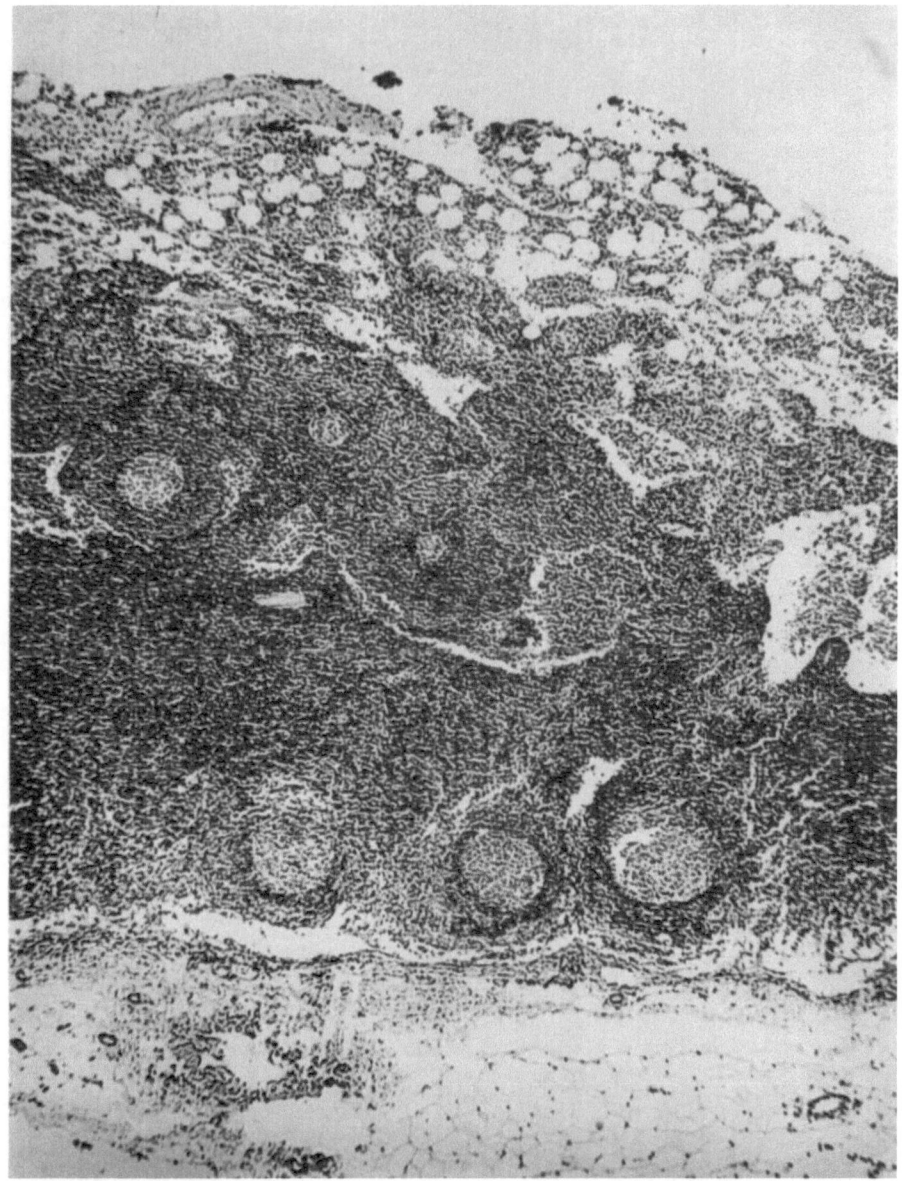

Fig. 1. Normal lymph node showing multiple germinal centers with active lymphocyte pro-liferation

the same changes seen in nodes of normal pregnancy. The nodes were obtained at autopsy. Neither patient received chemotherapy (Figs. 3 and 4).

B. HCG levels and total circulating lymphocytes

1. With the foregoing information it seemed logical to examine the total circu-

2*

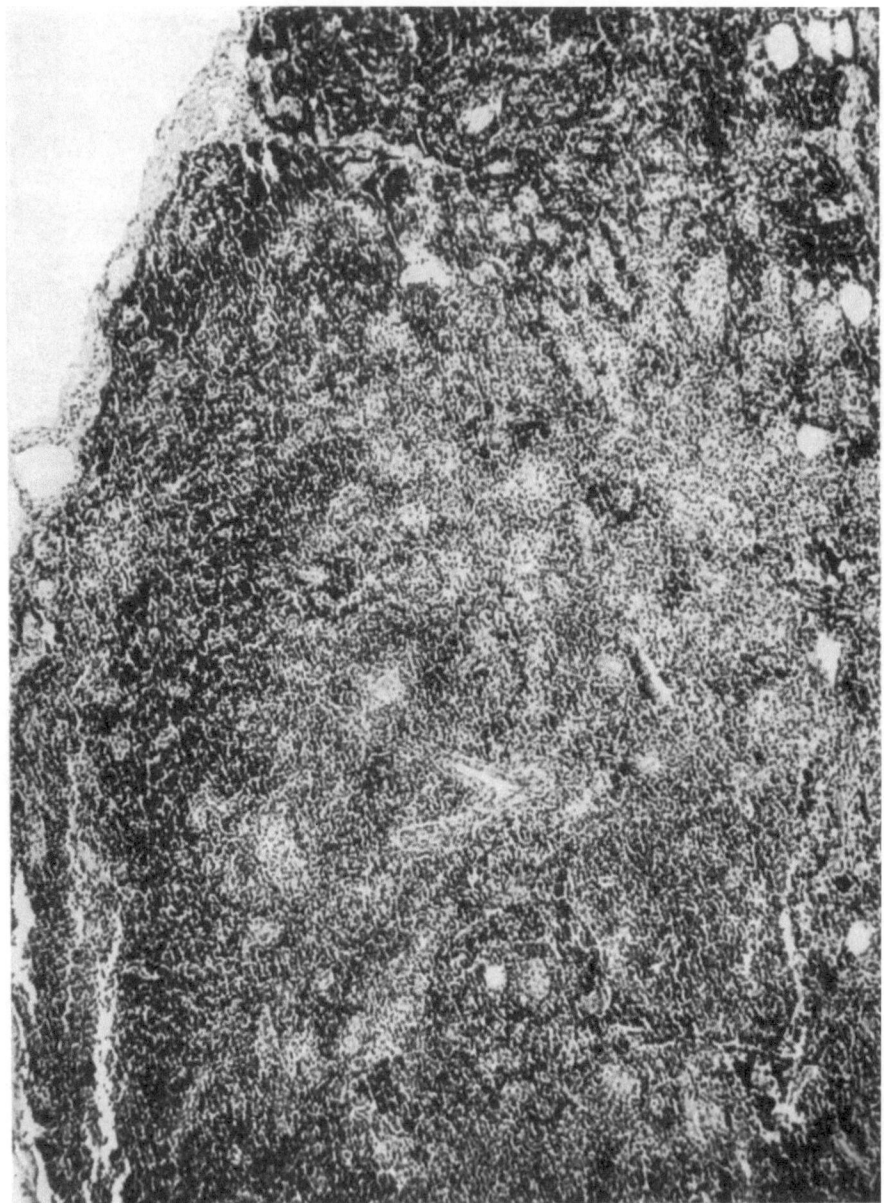

Fig. 2. Typical section from lymph node of normal term human pregnancy. The absence of germinal centers and increased reticulum is characteristic of lymph nodes from pregnant women

lating lymphocyte levels in choriocarcinoma retrospectively to see if they were depressed, and if so, to relate this to human chorionic gonadotropin (HCG) levels and to the clinical course. The absolute lymphocyte count was derived retrospectively by leukocyte count multiplied by per cent of lymphocytes in the differen-

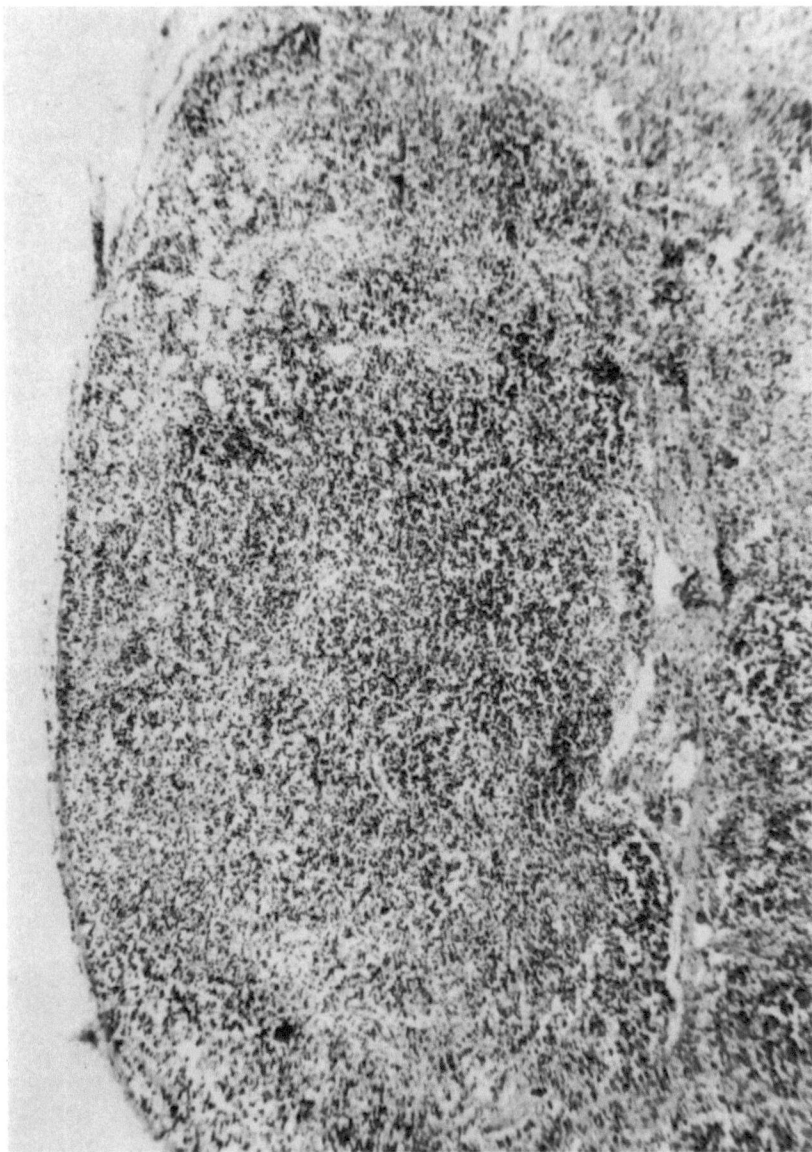

Fig. 3. Section of lymph node from a patient with choriocarcinoma showing complete absence of germinal centers. (×27)

tial count. The normal absolute lymphocyte count ranges from 1,500 to 3,000 lymphocytes/mm³.

2. Twelve case records made available to me from the Memorial Center proved satisfactory for analysis. The cases were abstracted and plotted as shown in Figs. 5, 6, and 7.

In summary, 11 out of 12 cases showed this kind of inverse relationship between the HCG titer and the absolute lymphocyte count. The lymphocyte levels were

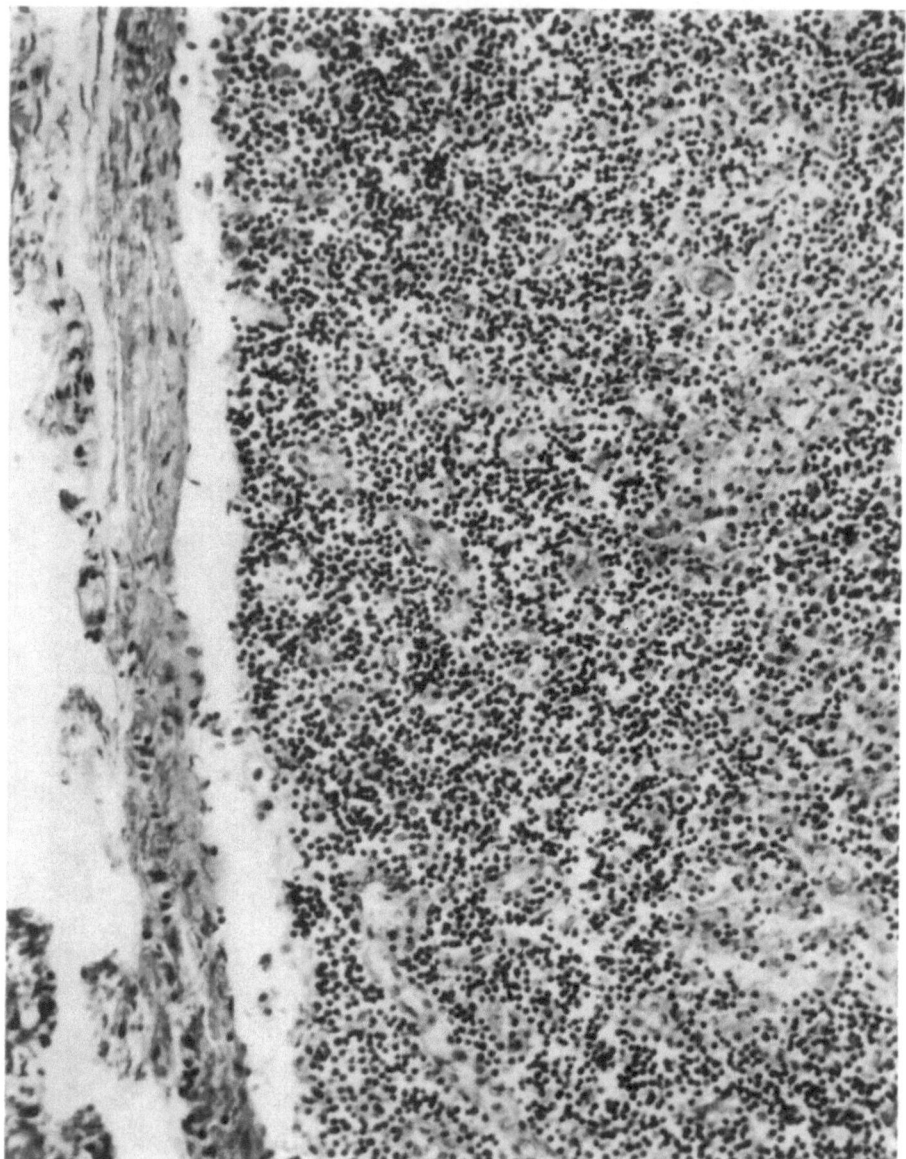

Fig. 4. Section from lymph node of patient with choriocarcinoma. No germinal centers are present. (×110)

below normal prior to the onset of therapy and either remained depressed if the patient did not respond or returned to normal if a clinical response did occur. There was an inverse relationship between the HCG titer and the absolute lympho-cyte count in all but one case and that case is shown in Fig. 7.

The potential importance of the findings are two-fold I think:

First, from a purely clinical point of view, the potential value to the clinician

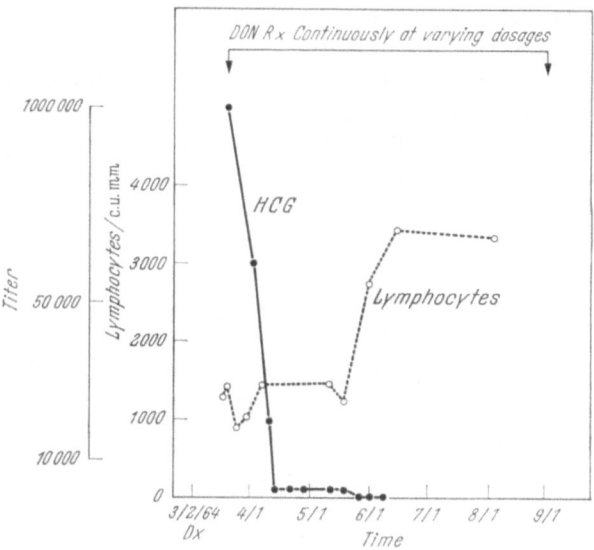

Fig. 5. The HCG titer dropped under DON therapy while the subnormal absolute lymphocyte count simultaneously held steady. When the HCG titer became undetectable the absolute lymphocyte count rose sharply to normal levels

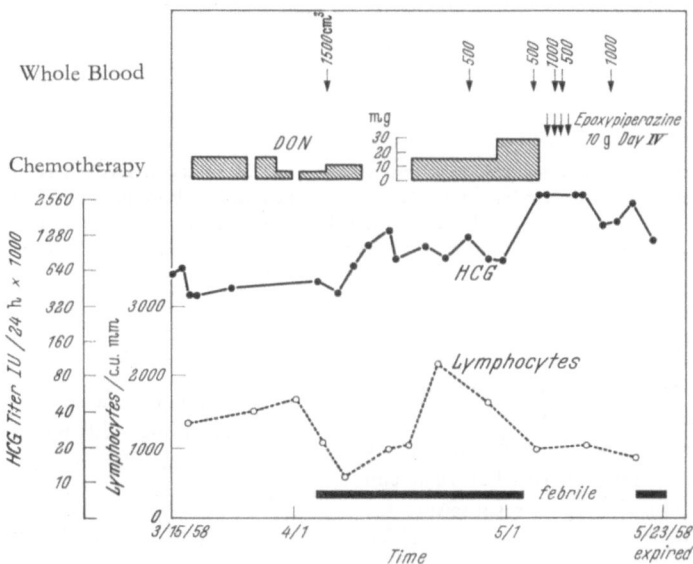

Fig. 6. A case of choriocarcinoma that failed to respond to therapy and expired. The HCG titer remained elevated throughout and the absolute lymphocyte count remained low throughout

is obvious. The use of the absolute lymphocyte count would be a far simpler method of following the response to chemotherapy than would human chorionic gonadotropin titers. It remains for those in areas where this disease is a frequent occurrence to take up this concept and test it thoroughly. The use of daily differential counts and white blood cell counts during therapy would, of course, be the first step in this analysis. From the cases shown I think it is obvious that the most striking change seems to occur in that affect some of the immune responses. If the lymphocyte is the mediator of homograft rejection either directly or indirectly, then perhaps therapy of choriocarcinoma bringing trophoblastic activity to a standstill allows the host immune responses to return to normal also.

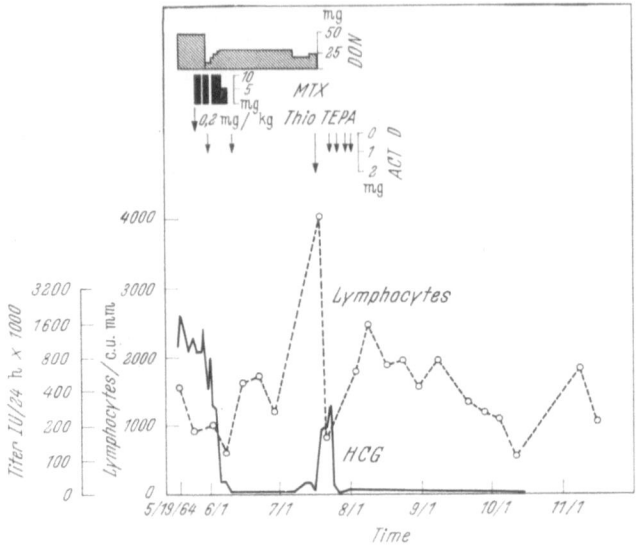

Fig. 7. The one case that was thought not to show the correlation. Even here there is a suggestion of a relationship between the HCG titer and the absolute lymphocyte count. On 7-15-64, the HCG titer rises and the lymphocyte level falls then at a time just before 8-1-64 the HCG titer falls and the lymphocytes return to normal levels. This represents the poorest correlation overall of the 12 cases analyzed

the very early phases of treatment and it is my impression that it is during this period when the lymphocyte count seems to have the most significance. Much more work must be done on this before it can be considered seriously as a substitute for HCG titer.

Second: This concept of the inverse relationship between the chorionic gonadotropin titers and absolute lymphocyte counts has theoretical implications of an immunologic nature. Trophoblast produces profound alterations in the endocrine system and it may be the secondary effects of these endocrinologic alterations

In summary

1. The known changes in the thymus and lymph nodes during normal pregnancy have been reviewed for animals and humans.

2. The findings in lymph nodes in choriocarcinoma (2 cases) have been demonstrated.

3. An apparent inverse relationship between the absolute lymphocyte count and HCG titers in cases of choriocarcinoma has been suggested. The possible significance and possible use of this finding have been discussed.

References

ADNER, M. M., SHERMAN, J. D., ISE, C., SCHWAB, R. S., and DAMESHEK, W., An immunologic survey of forty-eight patients with myasthenia gravis. *New Engl. J. Med.* 271, 1327—1333 (1964).

DOUGHERTY, T. F., and WHITE, A., Functional alterations in lymphoid tissue induced by adrenal cortical secretion. *Amer. J. Anat.* 77, 81—116 (1945).

HAMMAR, J. A., *Jb. Morph. mikr. Anat. Erg. Bd. ¿,* 498—503 (1926).

JOLLY, J., and LIEURE, C., Influence de la gestation sur la thymus. *C. R. Soc. Biol. (Paris)* 104, 451—454 (1930).

METCALF, D., The effect of thymectomy on the lymphoid tissues of the mouse *Brit. J. Haemet.* 6, 324—333 (1960).

NELSON, J. H., and HALL, J. E., Studies on the thymolymphatic system in humans. *Amer. J. Obstet. Gynec.* 90, 482—484 (1964).

NELSON, J. H., and HALL, J. E., Studies on the thymolymphatic system in humans. II. Morphologic changes in lymph nodes in early pregnancy and during the puerperium. *Amer. J. Obstet. Gynec.* 93, 1133—1136 (1965).

PERSIKE, E. C., Involution of thymus during pregnancy in young mice. *Proc. Soc. exp. Biol. (N. Y.)* 45, 315—317 (1940).

PLAGGE, J. C., Thymus gland in relation to sex hormones and reproductive processes in albino rat. *J. Morph.* 68, 519—545 (1941).

RATH, C. E., CATON, W., REID, D. E., FINCH, C. A., and CONROY, L., Hematological changes and iron metabolism of normal pregnancy. *Surg. Gynec. Obstet.* 90, 320—326 (1950).

Serial Passage of Choriocarcinoma of Women in the Hamster Cheek-Pouch

Roy Hertz

(with the technical assistance of Mr. Charles K. Turner and Mr. Howard L. Erwin)

Endocrinology Branch, National Cancer Institute, Bethesda, Md.

Greene (1952) initially described the survival and growth of human malignant tissue in the anterior chamber of the guinea pig's eye. These pioneer studies provided the basic experimental background for the observations to be reported here.

Subsequently, Toolan (1953) and Sommers et al. (1952) introduced the use of the hamster cheek-pouch as a site for such heterologous tumor transfer. They also found that the frequency of tumor takes could be very much increased by prior suppression of the immune response of the host animal. This was accomplished through x-irradiation or cortisone administration or through a combination of both of these proceedures.

Pierce et al. (1957) showed that certain human testicular tumors could be maintained as heterologous grafts by serial passage through similarly conditioned hamsters. They found that such tumors continued to produce the chorionic type of gonadotropin even after prolonged maintenance in the foreign host.

This report will describe the growth characteristics and hormonal behavior of seven strains of human uterine choriocarcinoma derived from metastatic tumor masses of seven women. The respective responses of these transplanted tumors to various chemotherapeutic agents will be compared with the response to these same agents previously observed in the individual donor patient. Certain immunological phenomena will also be described.

Materials and methods

Tumor tissue was initially obtained under aseptic conditions within one to seven hours after surgical excision or necropsy (Table).

Female golden hamsters of the NIH strain varying from one to three months in age were employed. Purina checkers were fed as a basal diet and a daily ration of kale, apples, and carrots was provided.

Under Nembutal anesthesia, each hamster received by direct inoculation into the cheek-pouch a piece of freshly excised tissue about 0.05 cu. cm. in volume. Recipient hamsters were either left totally untreated or they received 3 mgm of cortisone acetate in aqueous suspension at the time of inoculation and every third day for the ensuing two weeks. Repeated inspection of the everted cheek-pouch revealed the course of growth of the tumor inocula and this was recorded by a free-hand sketch of the size and shape of the growing tumor mass. Histological studies were performed on certain specimens by fixation in BOUIN's solution and staining with hematoxylin and eosin. Hamster plasma was prepared from heparinized blood drawn from the abdominal aorta under Nembutal anesthesia just prior to autopsy. Detailed observations were recorded at autopsy concerning the qualitative and quantitative

size and form of the tumors of treated and untreated control animals provided an estimate of the extent of inhibitory effects obtained (Fig. 1).

Upon discontinuing serial passage of each strain, portions of tumor were preserved in 50% saline and 50% glycerol

Table. *Seven strains of human choriocarcinoma in hamster cheek-pouch*

Strain	Date started	Source	Genera-tion[1]	Patient's clinical status
BO	7/22/57	Metastasis to breast (S)	132	Patient had incomplete remission on MTX; cerebral hemorrhage while off therapy; strain requires cortisone
WO	10/24/58	Brain metastasis (A)	216	Resistant to MTX after initial response.
MA	11/12/58	Lung metastasis (A)	140	Resistant to MTX after initial response.
JO	11/11/59	Lung metastasis (A)	118	Resistant to MTX after initial response; then noresponse to VLB or Cytoxan.
RE	1/21/60	Metastasis to cervix (S)	126	No chemotherapy before tissue obtained; subsequently had complete remission on MTX followed by Actinomycin D although still potentially responsive to MTX.
GR	11/2/60	Brain metastasis (A)	99	Limited response to MTX and VLB. Followed by resistance to both drugs.
CA	9/26/61	Lung metastasis (A)	46	No initial response to MTX or Actinomycin D.

(A) = Autopsy; (S) = Surgical specimen.

[1] As of Oct. 1, 1964 or prior to storage in liquid nitrogen and discontinuation of passage. All hamsters treated daily subcutaneously for 4 to 6 days beginning on day 7 after transplantation; effective doses were: (MTX) methotrexate — 50.0 mgm/kg; (VLB) Vinblastine — 0.75 mgm/kg; Actinomycin D — 50 gamma/kg.

effects of the tumor transplant on various endocrine organs.

All chemotherapeutic agents were administered daily subcutaneously in the form and dosage indicated in the legend of the Table. The drugs were started on the 6th day after transplantation when initial growth of the transplant could be clearly observed. Repeated sketches of the

under liquid nitrogen refrigeration. The frozen tissue from each strain was subsequently successfully reinoculated into untreated hamsters whenever required for further study.

Results and discussion

The seven successfully established strains of choriocarcinoma resulted from a total of thirty attempts. Five of these strains "took" initially in totally untreated hamsters and all but one strain can be maintained in such untreated animals. Cortisone conditioning has been continuously required for the transfer of one strain even after 132 passages over a period of seven years. However, this strain differs in no other observable feature from those maintained without cortisone.

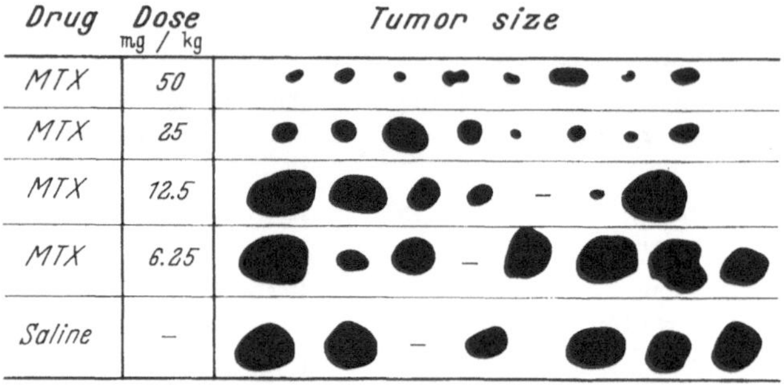

the same for previously frozen tissue as well.

Histological study of all strains reveals a close similarity in morphology of the transplant with that seen in the original human material. The rich vascularity of the tumor is very striking, the vascular elements and extravasated blood constituting about half of the tumor mass. Both cytotrophoblast and syncytiotrophoblast

Fig. 1. Effect of methotrexate on growth of choriocarcinoma

The growth behavior is essentially the same for all seven strains. The initial host response consists of the appearance within two to three days of a turbid exudate about the tumor inoculum. In the following three days this is rapidly replaced by highly vascularized, bluish-purple tissue which then extends and rapidly fills the cheek-pouch. In about 10 to 12 days the tumor reaches its maximum size of 1 to 1.5 cc. During the ensuing five to ten days the tumor loses its bluish color and becomes successively pink, grey and finally greenish yellow. At this point the necrotizing mass may slough and drain. Frequently, by 30 days following inoculation only a small residual scar may be found in the cheek-pouch. Less frequently the liquefied tumor mass is indefinitely retained.

Within 10 to 14 days after inoculation about 90% takes are observed and from 60 to 80% takes are already apparent after the first six days. The findings are

are clearly distinguished. In some preparations the syncytiotrophoblast is scant.

It is noteworthy that although this heterologously maintained tissue derives from tumor which is highly invasive in its natural host, no evidence of invasion of surrounding host tissue is observed in the hamster cheek-pouch. In addition, when the tumor is implanted subcutaneously, intraperitoneally or intracerebrally it grows at the site of implantation but has never been observed to invade or metastasize in a single one of the thousands of animals observed. The application of massive cortisone dosage has not altered its behavior in this regard.

GALTON et al. have described the chromosomal make-up of one of our tumor strains. The tumor is stated to "reveal an unstable and individually variable aneuploid karyotype. The modal chromosome number at the 56th passage was 80 and after an interval of nine months, at the 80th generation, it had risen to 88—92. However, there was no concomitant change in tumor histology" (GALTON et al., 1963).

WYNN and DAVIES (1964) have described the ultrastructure of this same tumor strain. Electron microscopy revealed cells which resembled normal syncytiotrophoblast in that the cytoplasm contained abundant endo-cytoplasmic reticulum, ribosomes and distinctive Golgi bodies. Distinctly cytotrophoblastic cells were also identified. In addition a type of transitional cell was described with structural resemblance in some features to both cytotrophoblast and syncytiotrophoblast.

Of major interest is the sustained hormonal activity of all of our tumor strains. From what is known of hormonal production by normal trophoblastic tissue the primary hormone to be expected would be chorionic gonadotropin. In addition thyreotropic hormone might be expected in view of the demonstrated association of hyperthyroidism with malignant trophoblastic disease and its suppression by oncolytic chemotherapy, as well as the presence of excessive quantities of thyreotropin in patient's plasma and tumor as demonstrated by biossay (ODELL et. al., 1963). Also the possible presence of placental lactogen as described in normal human placenta by ITO and HIGOSHI (1961) as well as by JOSINOVICH and MAC LAREN (1962) is to be considered in view of the frequency of persistent lactation in women with trophoblastic disease. The production of steroids related to the ovarian hormones may also be expected because of the synthesis of such substances by the normal placenta.

Thus, the intact female hamster bearing any of our tumor strains exhibits an extreme gonadotropic response consisting initially of extensive follicular stimulation which subsequently gives way to extensive luteinization. Although hemor-

rhagic follicles are frequently seen, ovulation is not observed. The uterus shows marked enlargement and hyperemia reflecting the ovarian hormonal response. These ovarian and uterine effects are seen in essentially the same degree in the hypophysectomized tumor-bearing hamster. However, no uterine effects are observed in the ovariectomized hamster indicating a lack of steriod-type hormone production.

The mammary glands of the intact tumor-bearing hamster are not grossly stimulated. However, detailed microscopic examination of such mammary tissue has not been carried out. Immunofluorescence study of the tumor tissue is also to be carried out since SCIARRA et al., (1963) have demonstrated the presence of a "growth hormone-prolactin" in normal syncytiotrophoblast through the application of specific fluoresceinized antiserum.

In the hypophysectomized hamster there is neither gross nor histological evidence of thyreotrophic effect or adrenocorticotrophic effect from the tumor. These negative observations apply equally to all strains despite the fact that our CA strain was derived at autopsy from a patient who had been freed of prior evidence of hyperthyroidism by oncolytic therapy (ODELL et al., 1963).

The distribution of the tumor-produced gonadotropin in the host's tissues has been repeatedly studied for several strains. This has been done by biossay of body fluids or tissue homogenates by either the rat ovarian weight assay or the mouse uterine weight assay. Fresh tumor homogenates contain about 50 I. U. per gm. Urine and blood contain about 20 to 30 I. U. per millilitre. It is, however, interesting that homogenates of liver, kidney, muscle and spleen contain no detectable biological activity. This indicates that although the hormone can be cleared by the kidney it does not readily enter the cells of peripheral tissues.

The ultimate rejection of the tumor by the host indicates a delayed immune response to the presence of heterologous tissue. Accordingly, we have found that a hamster which has previously rejected a tumor after several weeks growth is completely resistant to reinoculation for at least several months. Moreover, the daily injection of 2 ml of plasma from such a tumor-resistant animal will completely inhibit tumor growth in a previously untreated hamster. Hence both active and passive resistance to tumor inoculation may be demonstrated. However, prior exposure of hamsters to human serum globulin will also impart such resistance to tumor inoculation. This indicates that the resistance relates to the formation of species specific antibodies against antigens of human origin and regrettably not to tumor-specific antigens. This phase of induced resistance to tumor inoculation merits extensive study.

Another immunological aspect of these studies relates to the fact that chorionic gonadotropin is known to be specifically antigenic in numerous species. Antibodies to this hormonal antigen can be readily demonstrated by classical immunological methods as well as by neutralization of hormonal effects in bioassay. Accordingly, we have tested by bioassay the sera of animals having previously borne hormone-producing choriocarcinoma for evidence of such anti-hormonal activity. In no instance was such anti-hormonal activity demonstrable. Moreover, prolonged administration of massive doses of purified human chorionic gonadotropin to normal hamsters failed to yield anti-hormonal sera. Accordingly, it would seem that whereas the hamster shows good immune response to growing human choriocarcinoma as well as to human serum globulin, chorionic gonadotropin is not an effective antigen in this species.

The effect of a wide variety of drugs upon the growth of well established tumors during the second week following inoculation has been studied according to the procedures outlined above. We have done most extensive work with methotrexate. We were impressed at the outset by the remarkably high tolerance of the hamster for methotrexate. Such unusual resistance to the effect of colchicine had been previously described (Orsini and Paustry, 1952). Similarly, we found that the required dose for complete tumor inhibition was about 50 mgm per kilogram when administered daily subcutaneously on each of four consecutive days (Table). This represents about 100 times the dose found to induce clinical toxicity and tumor response in women. Nevertheless, in the hamster, this very high dosage produced no apparent systemic toxicity as manifested by loss of body weight, change in coat quality, diarrhea or ulceration of oral mucous membranes.

Profound tumor inhibition was uniformly observed in all seven strains of tumor in response to this dose of methotrexate (Fig. 1). It shold be emphasized that five strains originated from patients who had exhibited unequivocal evidence of unresponsiveness to previously effective doses of methotrexate (Table). This discrepancy may rest on the fact that in the experimental system we are testing the growth and survival of freshly transplanted tumor cells from a heterologous source whereas in the patient these same tumor cells are isologous and have been resident in the host for prolonged periods by the time drug resistance is encountered. That the quantitative difference in tolerated dosage between human and hamster is probably not a factor in the discrepancy is shown by the fact that the effective dose of the other drugs to be discussed below is comparable in man and hamster despite a similar discrepancy in responsiveness between the two species. This, then, is a good demonstration of the great fallibility of considering animal experimental data to be directly applicable to man despite certain broad similarities.

We have previously described the marked suppression of growth of these tumor strains produced by the Vinca alkaloids (HERTZ, 1960). In the case of vinblastine the effective and well-tolerated dose in the hamster (Table 1) closely approximated the effective but highly toxic dose in women (HERTZ et al., 1960). Moreover, this drug was effective in two strains of tumor which had been derived from patients in whom a prior therapeutic trial had induced no apparent tumor response.

Actinomycin D has similarly proven uniformly effective in inhibiting all seven tumor strains although one of these was derived from a patient who had proven totally unresponsive to this compound (Table).

In addition to the drugs just mentioned we have screened a wide variety of steroidal, alkaloidal and antibiotic preparations for possible inhibitory effect. The only significant inhibition observed not related to general systemic toxicity has been in the case of such alkylating agents as cyclophosphamide and in several preparations derived from podophyllotoxin. The activity observed in this latter group of agents warrants further investigation with a view to possible clinical trial.

In summary, it may be stated that (a) seven strains of heterologously transplanted human choriocarcinoma of fetal origin have been established through serial passage in the hamster cheek-pouch, (b) the endocrinological and immunological behavior of these tumors has been characterized, and (c) the usefulness of these tumor strains for chemotherapeutic explorations has been described.

References

GALTON, M., GOLDMAN, P. B., and HOLT, S., Karyotypic and morphologic characterization of a serially transplanted human choriocarcinoma. *J. nat. Cancer Inst.* **31**, 1019—1035 (1963).

GREENE, H. S. N., The significance of the heterologous transplant ability of human cancer. *Cancer (Philad.)* **5**, 24—44 (1952).

HERTZ, R., Suppression of human choriocarcinoma maintained in the hamster cheek-pouch by extracts and alkaloids of Vinca Rosea. *Proc. Soc. exp. Biol. (N. Y.)* **105**, 281—282 (1960).

—, LIPSETT, M. B., and MOY, R. H., Effect of vincaleukoblastine on metastatic choriocarcinoma and related trophoblastic tumors in women. *Cancer Res.* **20**, 1050—1053 (1960).

ITO, Y., and HIGASHI, K., Studies on the prolactin-like substance in human placenta. II. *Endocr. jap.* **8**, 279—287 (1961).

JOSIMOVICH, J. B., and MacLAREN, J. A., Presence in the human placenta and term serum of a highly lactogenic substance immunologically related to pituitary growth hormone. *Endocrinology* **71**, 209—220 (1962).

ODELL, W. D., BATES, R. W., RIVLIN, R. S., LIPSETT, M. B. and HERTZ, R., Increased thyroid function without clinical hyperthyroidism in patients with choriocarcinoma. *J. clin. Endocr.* **32**, 658—664 (1963).

ORSINI, M. W., and PAUSKY, B., The natural resistance of the golden hamster to colchicine. *Science* **115**, 88—89 (1952).

PIERCE, B., VERNEY, E. L., and DIXON, F. J., The biology of testicular cancer. I. Behavior after transplantation. *Cancer Res.* **17**, 134—138 (1957).

SOMMERS, S. C., CHUTE, R. N., and WARREN, S., Heterotransplantation of human cancer. I. Irradiated rats. *Cancer Res.* **12**, 909—911 (1952).

SCIARRA, J. J., KAPLAN, S. J., and GRUMBACH, M. M., Localization of anti-human growth hormone serum within the human placenta: evidence for a human chorionic growth hormone-prolactin. *Nature (Lond.)* **199**, 1005—1006 (1963).

TOOLAN, H. W., Growth of human tumors in cortisone-treated laboratory animals: the possibility of obtaining permanently transplantable human tumors. *Cancer Res.* 13, 389—394 (1953).

WYNN, R. M., and DAVIES, J., Ultrastructure of transplanted choriocarcinoma and its endocrine implications. *Amer. J. Obstet. Gynec.* 88, 618—633 (1964).

Synopsis of discussion I

Dr. KOSS remarked on the analogy of trophoblastic neoplasia with the evolution of carcinoma of the cervix where intra-epithelial carcinoma in situ is a less malignant neoplasm than invasive cancer of the cervix.

Dr. BILLINGHAM emphasized that the intimation of immunologic participation in rejection was circumstantial only, and resulted from observation of spontaneous regressions and responses to chemotherapy. It may be that the regression of trophoblastic neoplasia and of normal trophoblast occurs by similar mechanisms. Since there is no increase of tumors nor uncontrolled trophoblastic growth in isologous matings, immunologic defense would not appear to be critical. The trophoblast even though in direct contact with maternal blood has no apparent paternal antigens and therefore must be in and of itself a barrier, or be screened by a physical barrier from serving as an antigen to the mother. Dr. BURCHENAL noted that if trophoblast were non-antigenic it should transplant widely in other species. Six of 7 of Dr. HERTZ's transplanted choriocarcinomas do not require cortisone for maintenance in hamsters, whereas one does. Transplantation of human choriocarcinoma to the rat, however, is successful only if the animals are receiving corticosteroids and have been x-rayed. Transplantation into the uterine wall of hamsters prepared with x-ray, steroids and progesterone has been unsuccessful. Dr. HRESHCHYSHYN noted that in abdominal pregnancy in mice fibrinoid deposition between trophoblast and maternal tissues was found. Dr. HSU reported the transplantation of mole to hamster cheek pouch

and the recognition of normal villi in the first transplant generation.

Dr. NELSON could not exclude the possibility that the lymphopenia he observed was a characteristic of advanced cancer per se. Dr. BILLINGHAM commented that MEDAWAR had questioned whether anergy in pregnancy was caused by steroids. Homografts are accepted on day 24 of pregnancy in rabbits possibly because of anergy, but BILLINGHAM doubted that lymphopenia was sufficient to explain the phenomenon. NELSON questioned whether multiple factors weren't operative including lymphopenia, the low antigenicity of trophoblast, possibly because of a physical barrier, and perhaps local endocrine function of the trophoblast. Dr. BAGSHAWE cautioned against so gross an index of endocrinologic function as lymphocyte counts compared to the exquisite sensitivity of gonadotropin titrations.

Dr. BORJA reported that 3 women with choriocarcinoma treated with surgery and adjuvant chemotherapy, who had regression of their neoplasms and fall of gonadotropin titers to zero, rejected transplants of their husbands skin in 7 to 15 days. One patient whose pulmonary metastases did not regress and whose gonadotropin titer rose was tolerant of her husband's skin for one month. These observations suggest less importance of immunologic tolerance of the paternal antigens than of inability to respond appropriately when profoundly ill with advanced cancer.

Dr. ACOSTA-SISON has seen three hydatidiform moles with living fetuses and one choriocarcinoma with a live fetus. Thus the diseases are not primarily of the embryo, but of the trophoblast.

Trophoblastic or Chorionic Tumors as Observed in the Philippines

H. Acosta-Sison, M. D.

Department of Obstetrics and Gynecology, University of Philippines, Manila
Philippines

Trophoblastic or chorionic tumors are quite common among our poor Filipino women. This is one of the ailments we have in common with the poor women of Oriental countries, and I believe that the cause is a defective gene in the chromosome caused by a deficient diet which is low in protein content. Our poor eat mostly rice and vegetables and very little animal protein.

Incidence. In the Philippine General Hospital the incidence of the most common form of trophoblastic tumor, hydatidiform mole, is 1:200 pregnancies. In America and in Europe the incidence is 1:2,500—3,000 pregnancies.

Hydatidiform mole is an abnormal pregnancy wherein the chorionic villi are converted into cysts because of the liquefaction or degeneration of the mesodermic core of the chorionic villus. When its epithelial covering — the syncytiotrophoblasts or the syncytio- and cytotrophoblasts (Langhans cell layer) are proliferative and consist of several layers, then the mole can be recognized as malignant, and it can either perforate the uterine wall or metastasize by way of the circulation, and rarely by the lymphatics. The emboli may be deposited in any organ where they ultimately grow into either chorioadenoma destruens or choriocarcinoma.

Our records show that the most frequent target of first metastasis is the lungs, then the vagina. But when other organs are affected such as the brain, the liver, kidneys and spleen, the outcome has usually been fatal. When the metastasis is confined to the lungs, or vagina or broad ligament, and is recognized and treated early, recovery is possible.

In my studies on 620 cases of hydatidiform mole admitted to the Philippine General Hospital from 1945 to 1964, I have found that advanced age and pulmonary tuberculosis predispose a mole to become malignant.

When a hydatidiform mole develops in a woman past the age of 38 or when she has had a recent episode or presently is suffering from pulmonary tuberculosis, she should be followed for the possible later development of chorionic malignancy even though the biopsy of the mole is benign or Grade I. Pelvic examinations and quantitative determinations of chorionic gonadotropin in her urine should be repeated frequently for 6—12 months. Vaginal metastasis, uterine bleeding, subinvolution of the uterus or the presence of a pelvic mass are indicative or suspicious. Her chest should be submitted to X-ray examination for the presence of metastasis. In the absence of chorionic malignancy in the uterus, it should be completely involuted at the end of 6 weeks after curettage for mole or term delivery. Operation should not be delayed in cases of chorionic malignancy in the uterus. Early uterine chorionic malignancy may also be treated by methotrexate in young women when one wishes to preserve the uterus for child bearing.

Methotrexate, however, can be a very toxic drug. Before it is given, the kidneys and the liver should be normal. Methotrexate depresses the bone marrow and when toxic symptoms, such as stomatitis or rashes in any part of the body, or diminution of the red cell or white cell count, bleeding or diarrhea appear, the drug should immediately be discontinued.

I have termed certain clinical signs that point to the diagnosis of chorionic malignancy H B Es. H represents the history of having expelled a product of conception which can be a mole, an abortion or miscarriage, or even a term delivery. B refers to bleeding from the uterus. Es refers to enlargement (larger than normal) and softening of the uterus. The s is small because when the uterus is contracting, it may not be soft but hard. When H B Es is present it means chorionic tissue in the uterus. The tissue may be mole, invasive mole (chorioadenoma destruens) or choriocarcinoma. If not found to be mole by curettage (and subsequent correction of H B Es) the uterus should be removed in elderly women. In young women, who would like to have more children, leave the uterus and treat the malignancy with chemotherapy and watch the patient for the continuation of malignancy. Cure may be known by the absence of symptoms, complete involution of the uterus, negative X-ray findings in the chest, absence of any mass in the body, and negative gonadotropin test of the urine.

Chorioadenoma destruens

Pathologists abroad regard chorioadenoma destruens as a benign chorioma that does not metastasize. They admit, however, it can kill a patient through hemorrhage when it perforates the uterus. My experience in 41 cases of chorioadenoma destruens is that metastasis occurred in 11 cases or in 27 per cent; and in 10 cases or in 24 per cent, the uterus was perforated giving rise to intraperitoneal hemorrhage from 500—2,000 cc. Wei of Taiwan also had metastasis in 25 per cent of 12 cases. Prawirohardjo and associates of Indonesia also observed metastasis in 50 per cent of 10 cases. They call it "villous choriocarcinoma", and Novak terms chorioadenoma destruens as a "milder variant of chorioepithelioma malignum". From this opinion chorioadenoma destruens cannot be regarded as a benign chorioma.

Since chorioadenoma destruens can kill a patient because of hemorrhage, when present in the uterus, it should be treated immediately. For older women who do not want any more children, it would be best to perform panhysterectomy. The ovaries should not be removed unless they are affected.

For young women who would like to have more children, chemical treatment should be tried, preserving the uterus for future child bearing. The patient should, however, be closely watched for the continuation of malignancy.

Syncytial endometritis (syncytioma)

This is another form of chorionic pathology made up of syncytial cells which is universally regarded as benign. It does not perforate the uterus and does not metastasize. I have in my record 5 cases who because of uterine bleeding (2 after term delivery, 2 after abortion and 1 after mole) had the uterus curetted. The biopsy of uterine curettings was only syncytial endometritis, so nothing was done to the patients. All patients eventually died from chorionic epithelioma.

From the above experience despite negative biopsy in the curettings, I have learned to watch the patient for continuation of the bleeding which would dictate whether treatment should be given or not. [Syncytial endometritis may be indicative of endometrial response to trophoblastic neoplasia elsewhere. — Ed.]

One of the pathologic specimens I have seen was a chestnut-sized metastasis in half of the cerebrum which the pathologist called syncytioma because it was entirely made up of syncytial cells.

Choriocarcinoma

Choriocarcinoma is the most malignant form of cancer. From 1950 to 1962 we admitted 105 cases of choriocarcinoma to the Philippine General Hospital among 120,619 obstetrical cases. This shows an incidence of 1:1,382 pregnancies which is more than ten times the incidence of choriocarcinoma in Western countries which is 1:13,850 pregnancies as given by SCHUMANN and VOEGELIN.

The types of pregnancy that gave rise to these choriocarcinomas are as follows:

Hydatidiform mole: 63 cases or 60 %.

Early abortion: 24 cases of 23 %.

Term delivery: 11 cases or 10.4 %.

Concomitant with a
5 month living fetus: 1 case or 0.9 %.

Ab initio or primary
choriocarcinoma: 6 cases or 5.7 %.

Methods of Diagnosis

The demonstration of choriocarcinoma cells in the curettings of the uterus is the accepted scientific method. Unfortunately, not all cases of uterine choriocarcinoma can be diagnosed by the demonstration of malignant cells in the uterine curettings. When the malignant cells are in the myometrium beyond the reach of the curette, the biopsy of the uterine curettings will give a false negative report. In these cases, we have to rely on the clinical (HBEs) signs to dictate what should be done for the patient. In the presence of HBEs the uterus should be removed and in cases of choriocarcinoma both ovaries should also be removed. Usually in these cases the frog test of the urine will show high values of chorionic gonadotropin.

Symptoms: Abnormal bleeding from the uterus occurring a few days or weeks after the expulsion of the products of conception was the complaint of 82 patients (78 %). In these patients, the malignant growth was located in the endometrium. But in 23 cases (22 %) no abnormal bleeding occurred from 4 months to 2 years after the expulsion of the products of conception. Either spotting or profuse bleeding occurred at the end of this interval. In these cases, it was found that either the uterus was free from malignancy or the malignancy began at the myometrium with metastasis in other parts of the body such as the intestines, tissues surrounding the abdominal cavity, the lungs, spinal cord, or the brain. In the case where the spinal cord or the kidney was involved, the first complaint was back pain.

Because of its frequency, abnormal bleeding after the expulsion of the products of conception should be given importance in pointing out the presence of malignancy in the uterus.

Treatment: The treatment for chorionic malignancy is early surgery aided when indicated by other means. The drug that has given us the best result is methotrexate. This, however, can be a very toxic drug. Before its administration tests should be made for the normalcy of the liver and kidney. The red cell count should be adequate and the white cell count should be normal. They should be examined every 2—3 days while the drug is being given. And when signs of toxicity occur in the form of stomatitis, pink rashes over any part of the body, diminution of the red cell or white cell count, bleeding, or diarrhea — the drug should immediately be discontinued. If she is still harboring the growth the drug may be continued when she recovers.

We can tell if the patient is free from malignancy if she has no complaint, the X-ray of the chest is negative for meta-stasis, there is no mass in any part of the body, no uterine bleeding, and the urine is negative for chorionic gonado-tropin.

Of the 105 cases of choriocarcinoma, 30 recovered. Fifteen of the recovered cases had no metastasis. Thirteen of these cases were treated by panhysterectomy and bilateral salpingo oophorectomy. Two cases were treated only by methotrexate one with 95 mg. and one with 395 mg. before the urine became negative for chorionic gonadotropin. Fifteen cases showed metastasis. These were treated by surgery supplemented with methotrexate.

References

Acosta-Sison., Statistical study of 177 cases of hydatidiform mole in the Philippine General Hospital from April 6, 1945 to December 31, 1950. *J. Philipp. med. Ass.* 23, 652—660 (1951).
—, Is it really important to make an early diagnosis and treatment of hydatidiform mole? *Philipp. J. Surg.* 17, 180—183 (1962).
—, Observation which may explain the high incidence of hydatidiform mole in the Philippines and the asiatic countries. Congr. Int. de Gynecological D Obstetrique, Tome II p. 13 (Beauchenin, Montreal 1959).

Acosta-Sison., The relative frequence of various anatomic sites as the point of first metastasis in 32 cases of chorioepithelioma. *Amer. J. Obstet. Gynec.* 75, 1149—1152 (1958).
—, Influence of pulmonary tuberculosis on hydatidiform mole, *Obstet. Gynec.* 20, 103—106 (1962).
—, Chorioadenoma destruens; a report of 41 cases. *Amer. J. Obstet. Gynec.* 80, 176—179 (1960).
—, Is syncytial endometritis (syncytioma) always benign? *J. Philipp. med. Ass.* 39, 720—724 (1963).

The Natural History of Choriocarcinoma

DONALD P. C. CHAN, M. B., B. S., F. R. C. S. (Edin.), F. R. C. S. (Glasg.),
M. R. C. O. G., M. M. S. A. (Lond.)

*Professor and Head, Department of Obstetrics and Gynaecology,
University of Malaya, Malaysia*

Introduction

Choriocarcinoma is a malignant neoplasm of the embryonic chorion, both layers of the trophoblastic epithelium being involved. Microscopically, columns and sheets of anaplastic trophoblasts are seen invading the muscle and blood vessels in a lawless manner, haemorrhage and coagulation necrosis are constant features and villi are almost invariably absent. The uterus is certainly the commonest, but by no means the only, site where the primary growth is found. It characteristically metastasizes early and has a rapidly fatal course. Spontaneous regression has been observed, albeit rarely, in both uterine and extra-uterine lesions. This event is most probably due to the fact that choriocarcinoma, like the normal trophoblast, is not genetically identical with the host tissues and is therefore being treated as a homograft, immunity having been developed against it. Early surgery and chemotherapy have profound effect on the natural history of this very malignant neoplasm.

It was found by the Joint Project for Study of Choriocarcinoma and Hydatidiform Mole in Asia (1959) that choriocarcinoma does occur with extraordinary frequency in Asian countries. The incidence of choriocarcinoma was found to be 1 in 1,331 hospital deliveries in Hong Kong (CHAN, 1962), 1 in 1,382 pregnancies in a hospital practice in the Philippines (ACOSTA-SISON, 1962) and approximately 1 in 5,000 hospital deliveries in Singapore (TOW, 1964).

Age

It was also found by the Joint Project that the average age of Asian patients is older by statistical tests than that of American women, the figures being 33 and 28 years respectively. The average age of 40 cases of choriocarcinoma seen

Table I. *Age distribution in choriocarcinoma and parturient women*

	Chorio-carcinoma		Parturient women	
	No.	%	No.	%
Under 20	1	2.5	140	8.4
20—24	5	12.5	505	30.4
25—29	13	32.5	417	25.1
30—34	4	10.0	339	20.4
35—39	6	15.0	184	11.0
40—44	2	5.0	71	4.3
45—49	7	17.5	7	0.4
50	2	5.0	0	0
Total	40	100	1663	100

in Singapore between July, 1959 and October, 1964, over a period of 5 years and 3 months, was 33.8 years, the youngest patient being 17 and the oldest 50. Whilst it has been stated that most cases of choriocarcinoma occur in women under 35 years of age (HAINES and TAYLOR, 1962), 17 or 42.5 per cent of these 40 cases were 35 or more. Table I shows the distribution of cases according to the patent's age at the time of diagnosis of

nancies in the older age groups. The average number in the 17 cases aged 35 or more is 6.9 whilst that in the 23 cases under 35 is 4.3. Fig. 1 a and Fig. 1 b show respectively the distribution of cases by gravidity order in the 40 cases of choriocarcinoma and in the 1,663 women who serve as controls. These show a disproportionate frequency of choriocarcinoma in women who have had more than 4 pregnancies. This finding certainly sug-

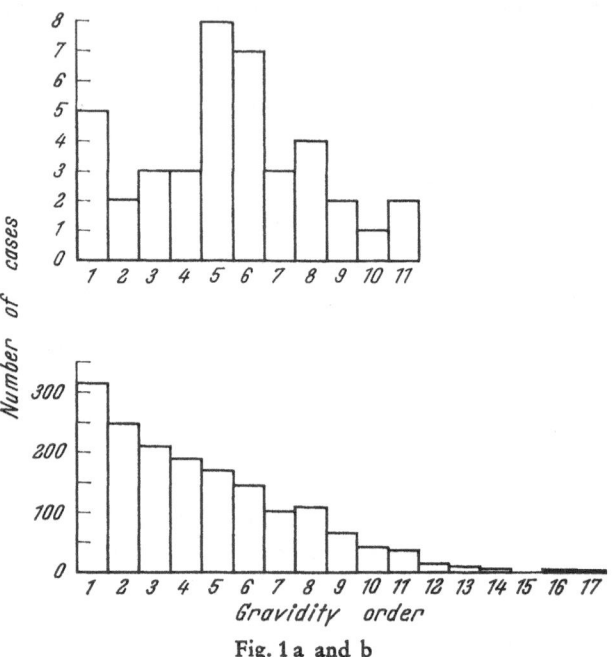

Fig. 1 a and b

choriocarcinoma. The maternal age distribution in 1,663 women who were delivered at Kandang Kerbau Hospital during the first 16 days of January 1963 is also shown. From these it can be seen that there is a tendency for choriocarcinoma to occur more frequently in the older age groups.

Parity: It was found by the Joint Project, too, that the average number of pregnancies among Asians (4.8 as against 2.4 among Americans) is consistently higher and that there are many more preg-

gests that a greater frequency of pregnancies may well be a causative factor (Fig. 1 a and Fig. 1 b).

It has been suggested by BARDAWIL and TOY (1959) that the survival of a choriocarcinoma in a patient may be the result of prior conditioning of the maternal soma by normal trophoblast. They quoted FLEXNER and JOBLING (1907) for having shown that the inoculation of rats with heat-killed tumor tissue appeared to enhance the proliferation of subsequently implanted viable fragments of the same growth. The showers of syncytial tropho-blast that become deported to the lungs during a normal pregnancy may serve a similar end by enhancing the growth of a later chorionic neoplasm. And it is to be expected that the larger the number of pregnancies the greater is the chance of deportation of trophoblast.

SCOTT (1962) analyzed 175 cases of choriocarcinoma registered at the Albert Mathieu Chorionepithelioma Registry, Chicago, and found that choriocarcinoma occurred with disproportionate frequency in first pregnancies. All but 17 of the 175 registry cases occurred within the United States. It was suggested, therefore, that every first pregnancy is a test of a wom-an's capacity to resist and control the invasive properties of the trophoblast produced by a particular mating and that having succeeded she is more or less im-mune to choriocarcinoma in the future, unless she takes a new mate to whose offspring she has not acquired resistance. This certainly has not been found to be true in Hong Kong and Singapore. One previous pregnancy only was found in 5 of the 40 cases studied (12.5 %), whereas 30, or 75 % had 4 or more previous preg-nancies.

Preceding pregnancy: According to HERTIG (1950), 50% of choriocarcinomas were preceded by mole, 25% by abortion, 22.5% by delivery and 2.5% ectopic pregnancy. PARK and LEES (1950), how-ever, pointed out that this distribution was only true when all cases diagnosed as choriocarcinoma were included and that if only fatal cases were considered the distribution was 32, 34 and 34 per cent respectively. They suggested that this difference indicated the tendency to over-diagnose choriocarcinoma following mole. In the present series, 27 (67.5 %) were preceded by a mole, 7 (17.5 %) by an abortion and 6 (15 %) by a delivery. If only the 24 fatal cases are considered, the

distribution is still 15 (62.5 %), 5 (20.8 %) and 4 (16.7 %) respectively. The latent interval between the previous pregnancy and the diagnosis of choriocarcinoma varied between 2 weeks and 7 years. It was six months or less in 11 of the 27 cases (40.7 %) which followed a mole and in 4 of the 13 cases (30.6 %) which followed an abortion or a delivery.

Clinical features: The symptoms of choriocarcinoma are well known, but unless thought of, the diagnosis is likely to be missed as the condition is relatively rare and may simulate many other gynaecolo-gical conditions (such as abortion and dysfunctional uterine bleeding), medical conditions (such as pulmonary tuberculosis and cerebro-vascular accident) and sur-gical conditions (such as bronchogenic car-cinoma and rupture of kidney, spleen and liver). The common symptoms are listed in Table II and it can be seen that they depend to a large extent on whether the growth is present in the uterus. Of the 40 cases of choriocarcinoma seen in Singa-pore, the growth was present in 22, and the correct diagnosis in them was un-doubted. The growth was absent in 18 uteri: this has been confirmed by examina-tion of the specimens removed at hyster-ectomy or postmortem in 14 cases and is presumed to be so in 4 cases who are still living and in whom hysterectomy has not been performed. Most probably no in-trauterine growth will be found in these 4 cases since all are menstruating normally without evidence of residual disease 1 year or more after the diagnosis of chorio-carcinoma.

Whilst symptoms relating to the genital tract (bleeding per vaginam and abdomi-nal pain) are almost invariably associated with the presence of a growth in the uter-us, respiratory symptoms (such as cough, haemoptysis, chest pain and dyspnoea) and cerebral symptoms (such as headache, blurring of vision and loss of consciousness) are relatively more common among cases where no growth is found in the uterus. In the latter group, amenorrhoea or oligomenorrhoea is sometimes a presenting symptom which is believed to be due to the effect of chorionic gonadotrophin on the ovaries leading to suppression of ovulation. Other rarer symptoms include abdominal swelling, pyrexia and anaemia.

There are altogether 24 deaths, the cause of which was cerebral haemorrhage in 15 (62.5 %), cachexia in 5 (20.8 %) and respiratory failure in 4 (16.6 %). An attempt was made to see if there is any correlation between the mortality rate and age, parity, the type of preceding pregnancy, the latent interval between the previous pregnancy and the diagnosis of choriocarcinoma, the presence or absence

Table II. *Presenting symptoms in patients with choriocarcinoma*

	Primary in uterus	Primary *not* found in uterus	Total
Number of cases	22	18	40
Pelvic symptoms			
Bleeding per vaginam	17 (77.3 %)	4 (22.2 %)	21 (52.5 %)
Abdominal pain	4 (18.2 %)	1 (5.5 %)	5 (12.5 %)
Amenorrhoea	0	5 (27.7 %)	5 (12.5 %)
Extra-pelvic symptoms			
Respiratory symptoms	8 (36.4 %)	10 (55.5 %)	18 (45.0 %)
Cerebral symptoms	8 (36.4 %)	7 (38.8 %)	15 (37.5 %)

On examination, the uterus was found to be normal in size in 22 cases and enlarged to the size of an 8 to 22 weeks' pregnancy in 18. Luteal cysts of the ovary were palpable in 3 and mestastases in the vagina and vulva were found in 8.

Pulmonary secondaries, as revealed by radiological examination of the chest, were found at one time or another in 31 (77.5 %) cases but they were invariably present in those who had died and on whom a postmortem had been performed.

Termination: Choriocarcinoma, whilst carrying a high mortality, is not inevitably fatal. Spontaneous regression may occur and a few authentic cases have been reported (Johnson, 1951; Hou and Pang, 1956), but it is definitely very rare. Localized lesions, however, may be cured by early surgical intervention. With the advent of chemotherapy, even cases with widespread metastases may be salvaged.

of growth in the uterus, and the use of chemotherapy. Thes results are shown in Table III.

(a) Whilst the incidence of malignant change in molar pregnancy increases with age (Tow, 1964), the mortality rate in choriocarcinoma is not related to age.

(b) Parity, however, increases not only the incidence of malignancy in molar pregnancy but also the mortality rate in choriocarcinoma

(c) Choriocarcinoma following molar pregnancy carries the best prognosis. This is to be expected and can be accounted for by the fact that women who have had a molar pregnancy are being carefully followed up. Any malignant change will, therefore, be diagnosed early and hence treated early.

(d) The mortality rate is three times higher in the group where the latent interval is 6 months or more than in that where it is less than 6 months. This may be accounted for partly by the fact that cases following a molar pregnancy have, on the whole, a shorter latent interval.

(e) The presence or absence of a growth in the uterus does not affect the mortality. The diagnosis in the 22 cases where a

(i) A left lower lung mass appeared $2^1/_4$ years after evacuation of a mole. It was accompanied by normal menstruation, persistently negative male toad test, and continual growth despite 4 courses of methotrexate. A wedge resection of the lung 8 months after appearance revealed

Table III. *Correlation between mortality rate and age, parity, preceding pregnancy, latent interval, primary in uterus and chemotherapy*

	No. of cases	No. re-maining alive	Mortality rate %
(a) Age			
Less than 35	23	9	60.8
35 and over	17	7	58.8
(b) Parity			
Gravida 1—4	13	6	53.8
Gravida 5—8	22	9	59.1
Gravida 9—11	5	1	80.0
(c) Prior pregnancy			
Mole	27	12	55.5
Abortion	7	2	71.4
Term delivery	6	2	66.6
(d) Latent interval			
Less than 6 mos.	15	11	26.6
6 mos. and more	25	5	80.0
(e) Primary in uterus			
Present	22	9	59.1
Absent	18	7	61.1
(f) Chemotherapy			
Without	16	4	75.0
With	24	12	50.0

growth is present is undoubtedly chorio-carcinoma. And so is the diagnosis in the 11 cases in whom the uterus is normal but death occurred as a result of dissemi-nated choriocarcinoma. The diagnosis of choriocarcinoma may, however, be queried in the 7 cases in whom no growth was found in the uterus (3 confirmed by hy-sterectomy and 4 suggested by the normal menstrual history with no evidence of residual disease) and who are still alive. How the diagnosis of choriocarcinoma was arrived at in these 7 cases is now briefly described below.

actively proliferating choriocarcinomatous cells. The patient is alive with no evidence of disease 2 years after the thoracotomy.

(ii) Four weeks after evacuation of mole a bluish nodule appeared in the va-gina which was excised and shown to be choriocarcinoma. She was treated with 5 courses of methotrexate and 6-mer-captopurine. Hysterectomy was perform-ed 9 months later and revealed a normal uterus. The patient is alive 3 years later with no evidence of disease.

(iii) Multiple pulmonary secondaries with haemothorax were detected 3 months

after evacuation of a mole. The patient
was treated with 11 courses of methotrexate till all lung opacities completely
disappeared. She became pregnant and
had a normal fulltime delivery 20 months
after evacuation. A solitary pulmonary
opacity appeared in the right upper lung
one month later. It increased in size at
first, remained stationary when methotrexate was restarted, but did not disappear. A wedge resection was performed.
Only fibrous tissue was seen on histological
examination and was thought to represent
a healed choriocarcinomatous lesion.

(iv) The other four cases, after evacuation of their molar pregnancies, had extensive pulmonary metastases upon which
the diagnosis of choriocarcinoma was based. Since no pathological material was
available, the correct diagnosis might well
be chorioadenoma destruens or malignant
mole or villous choriocarcinoma. [Gesta-
tional trophoblastic neoplasia, metastatic,
pulmonary, non-morphologic evidence,
antecedent molar pregnancy, morphologic
diagnosis uncertain. — Ed.] If this is the
case and if these four patients are excluded, then choriocarcinoma without a growth
in the uterus is associated with a higher
mortality than one with a uterine growth.

(f) Chemotherapy certainly has revolu-
tionized treatment and prognosis.

The uncorrected mortality rates for the
untreated and treated groups were 75 per
cent and 50 per cent respectively. But if
the 5 cases where the growth was confined to the uterus (4 in the untreated
and 1 in the treated groups) and the 2
cases which were admitted in the terminal
stage and died after only one course of
chemotherapy were excluded, then the
corrected mortality rates would be 100
per cent (all the 12 untreated patients
died) and 47.6 per cent (10 of the 21
treated cases died) respectively.

Discussion on sites of primary growth:
In choriocarcinoma, the commonest site
of the primary growth is undoubtedly the
uterus. But not infrequently, the uterus is
found to be normal and healthy and yet
definite choriocarcinomatous lesions are
present in the lungs and sometimes also in
the brain and other organs in the body.
There are 14 such cases in this series, not
counting the 4 cases in whom the diagnosis of choriocarcinoma cannot be definitely
confirmed. This interesting and indeed
common phenomenon is usually explained
on the assumption of spontaneous regression of the primary uterine growth which
apparently has been thought to be overcome by a local defensive mechanism. This
explanation is far from being satisfactory.
First of all, spontaneous regression is so
rare that it can hardly account for such
a common phenomenon. Secondly, there
is as yet no satisfactory explanation why
the defensive mechanism should be confined only to the uterus as it has been
shown by Hou and Pang (1956) that
distant "metastasis" is more extensive in
cases with no growth in the uterus. A more
likely explanation is that there is no primary choriocarcinomatous growth in the
uterus to start with and that the lesion in
the lung does not represent a secondary
metastasis from the uterus but that it
rather denotes a malignant transformation
of the trophoblasts which have been disseminated during the previous pregnancies,
be they hydatidiform mole, abortion or
fulltime delivery. This postulation is more
than supported by a careful study of the
first case summary and many other cases
that have been reported recently and cited
by Arias and Bertoli (1959) and Chan
and Pang (1964). The uterus had either
been removed or found to be normal and
healthy. There was usually an interval of
1 to 3 years between the preceding pregnancy and the appearance of the lung
lesion, but there was no reason why the
interval could not have been a short one.
The lesion was frequently solitary to start

with but in some was followed by widespread opacities which might represent secondaries from the primary choriocarcinoma in the lung.

It had been shown by ATTWOOD and PARK (1961) that trophoblastic emboli in the lungs were found in 43.6 per cent of their 220 woman dying during pregnancy or the puerperium. The ratio between 9 had their primary sites in the uterus and 4 in the lungs, giving a ratio of 9:4 or 100:44.4. This observation gives further support to the contention that most, if not all, cases where no growth is found in the uterus have their primary sites in the lungs. The fact that of the 23 cases which followed a molar pregnancy 10 had their primary sites in the lungs suggested

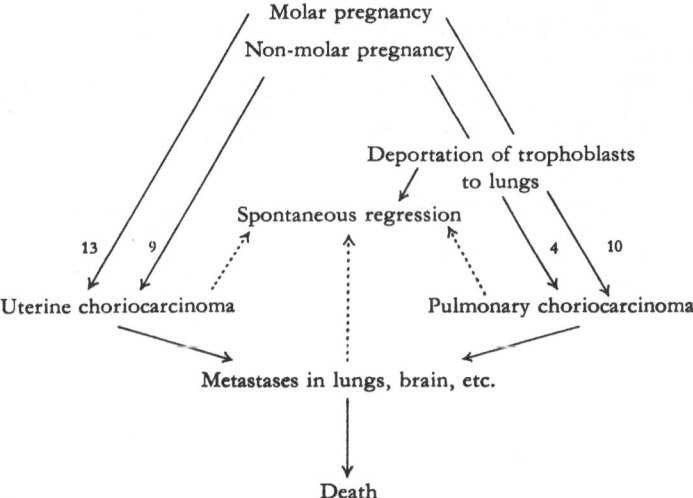

Fig. 2. Schematic presentation of natural history of choriocarcinoma

uterine choriocarcinoma and pulmonary choriocarcinoma might be expected to be 100:43.6 if one assumes that trophoblasts in the uterus and in the lungs have the same incidence of malignant transformation, which might even be due primarily to a breakdown of the maternal defensive mechanism. A postulated natural history of both these forms of choriocarcinoma is schematically presented in Fig. 2. Of the 13 cases of choriocarcinoma which followed an abortion or fulltime delivery, that trophoblastic deportation was a much more common occurrence during molar pregnancy.

Acknowledgement

I would like to express my thanks to Dr. S. H. Tow for his permission to report.

This work was accomplished while the author was Sepior Lecturer in Obstetrics and Gynaecology, University of Singapore.

References

ACOSTA-SISON, H., Studies in choriocarcinoma from 88 patients admitted to the Philippine General Hospital from 1950—1961. *Acta med. philipp.* 19, 2, 77—83 (1962).

ARIAS, R. E., and BERTOLI, F., Metastatic choriocarcinoma without primary lesion. *Obstet. Gynec.* 13, 737—740 (1959).

Attwood, H. D., and Park, W. W., Embolism to the lungs by trophoblast. *J. Obstet. Gynaec. Brit. Cwlth.* **68**, 611 (1961).

Bardawil, W. A., and Toy, B. L., The natural history of choriocarcinoma: Problems of immunity and spontaneous regression. *Ann. N. Y. Acad. Sci.* **80**, 197—257 (1959).

Chan, D. P. C., Choriocarcinoma. A study of 41 cases. *Brit. med. J.* **1962** II, 953—957.

—, and Pang, L. S. C., Late solitary pulmonary choriocarcinoma following hydatidiform mole. *J. Obstet. Gynaec. Brit. Cwlth.* **71**, 192—197 (1964).

Flexner, S., and Jobling, J. W., On the promoting influence of heated tumour emulsions on tumour growth. *Proc. Soc. Exp. Biol. (N.Y.)* **4**, 156—157 (1907).

Haines, M., and Taylor, C. W., The chorion. In: *Gynaecological Pathology*, p. 294—306, Boston: Little, Brown 1962.

Hertig, A. T., Hydatidiform mole and choriocarcinoma. In: *Progress in Gynecology*, edit. by Meigs, J. V. and Sturgis, vol. 2, p. 372—394 New York: Grune & Stratton 1950.

Hou, P. C., and Pang, S. C., Choriocarcinoma: an analytical study of 28 necropsied cases, with special reference to the possibility of spontaneous regression. *J. Path. Bact.* **72**, 95—104 (1956).

Johnson, W. R., Spontaneous and complete regression of extensive pulmonary metastases in a case of chorioepithelioma. *Amer. J. Obstet. Gynec.* **61**, 701—704 (1951).

Joint Project for Study of Choriocarcinoma and Hydatidiform Mole in Asia. Geographic variation in the occurrence of hydatidiform mole and choriocarcinoma. *Ann. N. Y. Acad. Sci.* **80**, 178—196 (1959).

Park, W. W., and Lees, J. C., Choriocarcinoma. A general review, with an analysis of 516 cases. *Arch. Path.* **49**, 73—104, 205—241 (1950).

Scott, J. S., Choriocarcinoma. Observations on the etiology. *Amer. J. Obstet. Gynec.* **83**, 185—193 (1963).

Tow, S. H., Choriocarcinoma. *J. Int. Fed. Gynaec. Obstet.* **2**, 111—124 (1964).

Early Development of Choriocarcinoma*

John I. Brewer, M. D., Ph. D., and Albert B. Gerbie, M. D.

Albert Mathieu Chorionepithelioma Registry American Association of Obstetricians and Gynecologists, and the Department of Obstetrics and Gynecology, Northwestern University Medical School and Passavant Memorial Hospital, Chicago, Illinois, U. S. A.

Albert Mathieu Chorionepithelioma Registry data

Age. Tabulation of the ages of the patients with trophoblastic disease registered in the Albert Mathieu Chorionepithelioma Registry is presented in Table I. The patient material is received from all parts of the United States but not all material is sent to the Registry. None has been sent on the basis of the age of the patient. In all probability this sampled data of age distribution is valid for all patients with trophoblastic disease in the United States.

In the patients 40 years of age and older hydatid mole occurred in 20 (6.7 %), chorioadenoma destruens [invasive mole-Ed] in 14 (16.6 %), and choriocarcinoma in 30 (11.7 %).

Race. In gathering data according to race only those patients residing in the United States and whose records were adequate were included. The distribution of 552 patients was as follows: Caucasian, 469; Negro, 66; Spanish American, 8; American Indian, 4; Japanese American, 2; Japanese Hawaiian, 2; Korean American, 1.

Gravidity. There were 609 patients whose records were adequate to evaluate the frequency of trophoblastic disease as a complication of the first or subsequent pregnancies (Table II).

When trophoblastic disease occurred during the first pregnancy (219 cases) the distribution by disease categories was: hydatid mole, 101 patients (46.1 %); chorioadenoma destruens, 31 (14.2 %); choriocarcinoma, 87 (39.7 %).

When trophoblastic disease occurred as a complication of the second or subsequent pregnancies (390 cases) the distribution was: hydatid mole, 181 patients (46.4 %); chorioadenoma destruens, 48 (12.3 %); choriocarcinoma, 161 (41.3 %).

Cook Country Hospital data

Cook County Hospital, Chicago, cares for the indigent patients in the County of Cook. Since the patients are all of the low socioeconomical group, are restricted to a small geographic region, are in such large numbers, and are managed in a single hospital, the data on the incidence of trophoblastic disease are of interest. To

* This study was supported by the United States Public Health Service Grant Ca 06616-01 and 02 from the National Cancer Institute and the Robert C. Ziebarth Educational and Training Fund.

Table I. *Age distribution in trophoblastic disease. 635 patients*.*
(Albert Mathieu Chorionepithelioma Registry)

Age (years)	Hydatid mole	Chorioadenoma destruens	Chorio-carcinoma
Under 20	46 (15.6 %)	18 (21.4 %)	24 (9.4 %)
20—24	100 (33.9 %)	18 (21.4 %)	71 (27.7 %)
25—29	82 (27.8 %)	19 (22.6 %)	62 (24.2 %)
30—34	30 (10.2 %)	11 (13.1 %)	39 (15.2 %)
35—39	17 (5.7 %)	4 (4.8 %)	30 (11.7 %)
40—44	10 (3.4 %)	7 (8.3 %)	15 (5.9 %)
45—49	5 (1.7 %)	5 (6 %)	12 (4.7 %)
50+	5 (1.7 %)	2 (2.4 %)	3 (1.2 %)
Total patients	295 (100 %)	84 (100 %)	256 (100 %)

* The numbers of patients in each category are not valid for the relative frequency of hydatid mole, chorioadenoma destruens and choriocarcinoma in the United States. Considerable selection is made by doctors in referring patients to the Registry. Those with choriocarcinoma are more apt to be referred.

Table II. *Trophoblastic disease complicating the first or subsequent pregnancies. 609 patients.*
(Albert Mathieu Chorionepithelioma Registry)

Age	No. of patients	As compli-cation of first pregnancy	As complication of second or subsequent pregnancy
Under 20	86	73	13
20—24	181	81	100
25—29	154	40	114
30—34	76	13	63
35—39	51	5	46
40—44	31	4	27
45—49	20	1	19
50+	10	2	8
Total No. pts.	609	219 (35.9 %)	390 (64.1 %)

the obstetric service there are an average of 23,000 pregnancies admitted annually. The data shown in Table III were kindly furnished by Dr. Agusta Webster, Chief of the Obstetric Service, Cook County Hospital.

Natural history: Early development of choriocarcinoma

Our knowledge has been very incomplete of the histologic features that characterize the early developmental stage of choriocarcinoma since but few cases have been observed. In the previous three that have been observed the basic feature of malignant trophoblastic change associated with villi within the normal placenta was evident but many of the accompanying changes in the progressive development of this lesion were not identified. In two of devoid of myometrial invasion and both patients died of widely disseminated choriocarcinoma. The latter rather convincingly indicates the lesions to be choriocarcinoma even though the usually accepted criteria for the diagnosis of this neoplastic lesion are not all fulfilled.

Table III. *Trophoblastic disease incidence at Cook County Hospital Chicago, Illinois. January 1, 1959 to December 1, 1964*

Total pregnancies

112,181	Women delivered (20 weeks' gestation and over)
25,959	Abortions (under 20 weeks' gestation)
138,140	Total pregnancies

Racial distribution

19,864	Caucasian	(14.38%)
118,276	Negro	(85.62%)

Number of patients with trophoblastic disease according to race

12	Caucasian	(16.9%)
59	Negro	(83.1%)
71	Total no. of patients	

Types of disease and incidence

Hydatid mole   66 (1 : 1,699 deliveries; 1 : 2,093 pregnancies)
(5 progressed to chorioadenoma destruens — 7.6%)
(2 progressed to choriocarcinoma —3%)

Choriocarcinoma

5	subsequent to pregnancy not of molar type
2	subsequent to molar pregnancy
7	(1 : 16,026 deliveries; 1 : 19,734 pregnancies)

All trophoblastic disease

71   (1 : 1,580 deliveries; 1 : 1,946 pregnancies)

the cases (DRISCOLL, 1963; McKELVEY, personal communication) a tiny region of choriocarcinoma was identified within the normal, term placenta. There was no myometrial invasion and there were no metastases. Both patients survived without therapy. In a third case (McKELVEY) a tiny lesion within the normal placenta was found, no invasion of the myometrium was observed, but the patient died of a widespread metastatic choriocarcinoma.

In the two additional cases to be reported here, the lesions were small, were located within the normal placenta, were

The characteristics in the early development of choriocarcinoma to be shown are the location of the lesion in the intervillous space, lack of invasion into the endometrium and myometrium, hyperplasia and anaplasia of the trophoblast, origin of the lesion in normal vascularized villi, spontaneous regression of portions of the malignant trophoblast, degeneration and loss of the formed villi during the development stages, invasion of the villus by its own trophoblast, lack of invasion and destruction of the fetal capillaries of the villi by the immediately adjacent malignant trophoblast, and absence of maternal tissue response as indicated by lack of accumulation of maternal lymphocytes, leukocytes and plasma cells in the region of the malignant lesion.

Case I (CR 388). At 24 weeks' gestation this patient had bleeding from a vaginal lesion, which upon biopsy consisted of trophoblast. One week later metastatic lung lesions appeared.

Both ovaries, tubes and the uterus containing a normal living fetus were removed. Grossly and microscopically no lesion was identified in the normal placenta or uterus.

Two weeks later the patient died. Autopsy revealed metastatic choriocarcinoma in the brain, lungs and vagina.

Because of these findings a renewed search for the primary lesion was made of the placenta and uterus. After some effort a 1 cm lesion was found microscopically within the normal placenta.

Histopathology of the placenta. Histologically, normal villi covered with normal trophoblast characteristic of this stage of gestation completely surround the region of abnormal trophoblast. The villi with abnormal trophoblastic proliferation have normal stromal elements and contain normal vascular structures in which fetal blood cells are present. Irregular large masses of syncytium and cytotrophoblast project into the intervillous spaces from both the tips and surfaces of the non-anchoring type villi. Both types of cells have immature characteristics and are deeply basophilic. Anaplasia is marked, some nuclei being huge. Normal and abnormal mitosis are numerous in the cytotrophoblast. Lacunae are present in the syncytial masses and in some regions these are so abundant and large that a lacy, spun-out appearance is created.

Degenerative changes (necrosis) are abundant within many of the masses of trophoblast in the intervillous space. Ear-

ly degeneration of the central villous core is observed at the edge accompanied by loss of the basement membrane. More extensive degeneration of the villous core involving the entire tip of the villus and accompanied by necrosis of its trophoblast is a frequent finding. The remaining portion of such a villus has an intact non-degenerated core with intact fetal capillaries that contain fetal blood and with non-degenerated trophoblast on its surface. Nearly complete necrosis of the central core and the overlying hyperplastic trophoblast, a further stage in the degeneration of the formed villus, is observed frequently. There is meager infiltration of leukocytes, lymphocytes and plasma cells. Degenerative changes are present in a mass of trophoblast lying within the lumen of a vein in the myometrium. These degenerative changes are spontaneous since the patient had received no therapy prior to the time these tissues were obtained.

In some of the masses of malignant trophoblast are small fetal capillaries that contain fetal erythrocytes. There are no villous stromal elements interposed between the trophoblastic cells and the fetal capillary endothelium. Despite this intimate contact there is no evidence of degeneration of the fetal endothelial cells and no invasion of the fetal capillary structures is observed.

No invasion by the malignant trophoblast of the stroma of the central core of its own villus was noted in the numerous sections studied.

One venous sinus, located at the myometrial-endometrial junction immediately beneath the localized placental lesion, contains a mass of abnormal trophoblast devoid of a formed villous structure.

Deeper in the myometrium, several venous structures contain masses of malignant trophoblast and others contain normal, formed villi encompassed by a thin layer of normal trophoblast.

In the autopsy material all the metastatic lesions are typical of choriocarcinoma with hemorrhage, necrosis and inflammatory cells and without formed villi. There is no direct invasion of the myometrium at any point.

The diagnosis was a small localized choriocarcinoma in an otherwise normal 26-weeks, placenta with multiple distant metastases.

Case 2. (N. U. M. S. 17632). In this patient, who was delivered of a living infant at term, there was partial involvement of the placenta with choriocarcinoma. Shortly after delivery roentgen study revealed multiple pulmonary metastatic lesions. Two weeks after delivery a curettage was performed and the diagnosis of choriocarcinoma was made. Death due to disease occurred shortly thereafter.

Histopathology of the placenta. The villi in the portion of the placenta uninvolved with choriocarcinoma contain normal stromal and vascular elements and have the usual narrow layer of syncytium covering their surfaces. The vascular structures contain fetal blood elements.

Within the placenta and adjacent to these normal villi is the choriocarcinomatous lesion in which the syncytial and cytotrophoblastic changes are typical of choriocarcinoma. There is marked hyperplasia and anaplasia and in the cytotrophoblast there are numerous normal and abnormal mitoses. The basophilia is intense. The trophoblastic growth is seen to originate from all surfaces of multiple formed villi of varying sizes and it projects into the intervillous space.

These villi giving rise to choriocarcinoma (Fig. 1) have the normal structural form of term villi; the stromal cells in the central core have the normal configuration and staining qualities; and the fetal capillaries are intact and filled with fetal blood cells. They differ from normal villi

only in that the covering trophoblast has malignant characteristics.

A striking feature is the degeneration in both the malignant trophoblast and the stroma of the formed villi.

In the malignant trophoblastic masses still residing within the confines of the placenta and still attached to the surface of the formed villi there are small regions of necrosis involving both the syncytium and the cytotrophoblast. In some locations the necrosis involves most of the mass of trophoblast. In these particular sites the stromal cores of the villi may show no evidence of degeneration and the fetal vessels are intact and filled with blood. In other regions the changes are more extensive and involve both the trophoblast and stromal elements of the villi. In numerous regions a villus contains a normal central core with malignant trophoblast on its periphery while in the portion at the tip the stroma has undergone necrosis and the surrounding trophoblast has been lost. Further along in the degenerative process "ghosts" of formed villi with "ghosts" of the attached malignant trophoblast are seen. Still more advanced are the regions in which only pink eosin stained amorphous material is present. In some of the villi "ghosts" the entire central fetal blood vessels are still intact and still contain blood cells. In rare instances the fetal vessels are filled with amorphous material. There is scant infiltration of maternal leukocytes and lymphocytes in these regions of degeneration. This is quite in contrast to the marked infiltration that is present in those metastatic trophoblastic masses that evidence necrosis and are located within maternal myometrial blood vessels.

Invasion of stroma of the central core of the villus by its own malignant trophoblast does occur but is not a prominent finding. Careful search is required to identify such instances. The basement membrane of one region of the villus has been lost and there are two small masses of trophoblast amidst the stroma of the central core. In a mass of malignant trophoblast surrounding fetal capillaries only a strand of stroma is interposed between,

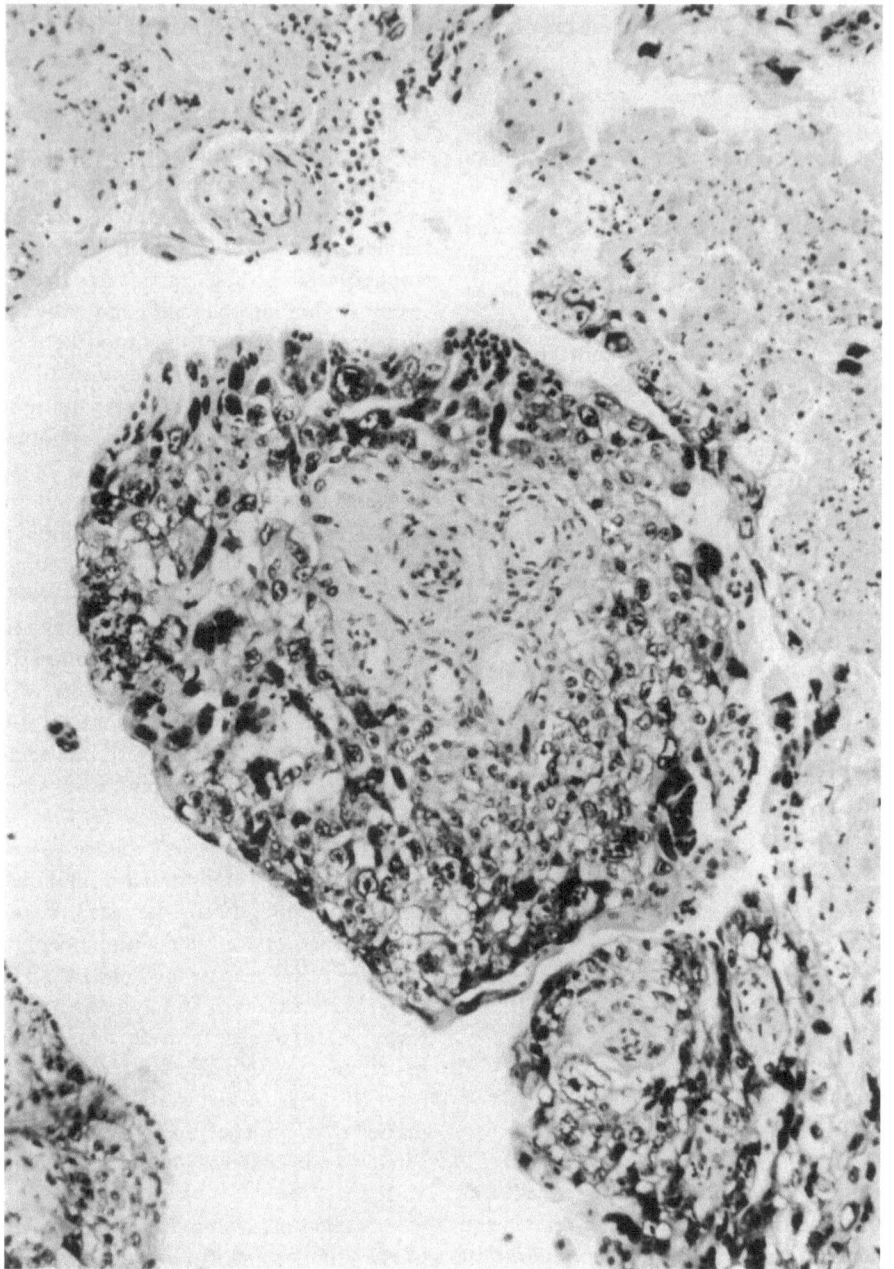

Fig. 1. Choriocarcinoma arising from a normal, vascularized term villus which is located within a portion of the normal placenta. The infant was born alive and well. The mother died of metastatic choriocarcinoma

and immediately adjacent are isolated strands of stroma scattered amongst the trophoblastic cells. In some regions the fetal capillaries, devoid of stroma, lie within the trophoblastic mass, the cells of which are in close approximation with the endothelium. The capillary is intact and contains a single column of fetal red cells. In serial sections this particular capillary is traced to its source which is a larger capillary within the stroma of a formed villus. While there is no stroma surrounding this capillary and while the malignant trophoblastic cells are in contact with the endothelium, there is no evidence of destruction of the fetal endothelial cells or of invasion of the fetal vessel. In no instance did we find this taking place. This phenomenon is in marked contrast to the profound and random destruction of the maternal endothelium and invasion of the maternal vessels observed in the process of normal implantation and in the regions of metastasis of choriocarcinoma in the myometrium and other sites.

The masses of choriocarcinoma in the uterine wall in this specimen are located within myometrial vessels. In some of these, local destruction of the endothelium has been replaced by a row of malignant trophoblastic cells in a manner similar to that which takes place in a normal implantation.

Comments

The observations of special interest in these early developmental stages of choriocarcinoma are: the origin of the lesion in normal placental villi and its location within the confines of the intervillous space; the spontaneous regression of portions of the malignant trophoblast and the stromal villous core and the scant infiltration of leukocytes and lymphocytes associated with this reaction; the

invasion of the stromal core of the villus by its own malignant trophoblast; and the loss of the formed villous structure during the developmental stages of choriocarcinoma.

1. The origin of choriocarcinoma in normal villi. It must be apparent to everyone that villi are present during the early developmental stage of all cases of choriocarcinoma that arise as a complication of pregnancy unless the presumption is made that the disease arises in the previllous trophoblast. Evidence for the latter is meager. That the former is true is borne out by the observations in all five of the early stages of the disease as described by DRISCOLL, by McKELVEY and by us in this report.

In the early inception of the disease only a few villi are involved. They lie adjacent to or may be surrounded by villi with normal trophoblast characteristic of the stage of pregnancy. The malignant trophoblast emanates from all surfaces of the villi. The stroma and the vascular structures of these villi are normal histologically. Villi so involved are of the unattached (non-anchoring) type in the five specimens studied. As a consequence of these relationships the malignant trophoblastic masses project into the intervillous space, not directly into the endometrium and myometrium. From this site, where they are completely surrounded by maternal blood, the fragmented masses extend directly into endometrial an/or myometrial veins. These phenomena are demonstrated in Case 1 (CR 388) and Case 2 (N. U. M. S. 17632) and undoubtedly occurred in the case observed by Mc KELVEY. In all three, a search of the placenta and the entire uterus disclosed the lesion within the placenta but failed to reveal any lesion in the endometrium or directly in myometrium. These three patients died with widely disseminated vascular metastasis.

4*

No dissemination of disease beyond the confines of the placenta and intervillous space was noted in the other early cases studied by Driscoll and by Mc Kelvey and these patients survived without therapy.

Thus, in the early stages of development choriocarinoma arising in a placenta not of molar type is a lesion located completely within the maternal circulating blood stream (the intervillous space). All five cases studied demonstrate this feature. In this position the malignant trophoblast is not in contact with maternal endometrial or myometrial tissue but is in direct contact only with maternal blood. In early lesions, then, only the maternal blood constituents circulating in the intervillous space have an opportunity to express defensive mechanisms to the progression of the disease. Not until later stages when the malignant trophoblast invades the tissues directly do the phenomena of tissue defense come into play as occurs in the normal implantation mechanisms associated with anchoring villi. While both normal implantation and trophoblastic diseases have been likened to a homograft reaction, there is obviously some dissimilarity in choriocarcinoma arising in a normal placenta. In the latter the "graft" of malignant tissue, if one may use the term, is not placed directly into the tissue but is suspended free in the maternal circulation. In normal pregnancy the "graft" is placed directly into the tissues of the host. This difference may have some pertinent but as yet unknown significance.

Spontaneous regression of portions of the malignant trophoblast and formed villi. In both specimens (CR 388 and N. U. M. S. 17632) there were varying degrees of degenerative changes in portions of the malignant trophoblast and villi in their primary site within the placenta. This was a spontaneous reaction since neither patient had received therapy.

In some regions entire masses of formed villi and malignant trophoblast have simultaneously undergone complete degeneration.

A striking feature in the necrosis of the malignant lesion within the placenta is the relative absence of maternal leukocytes and lymphocytes. This is in marked contrast to the abundant infiltration of such cells in the masses of malignant trophoblast, portions of which have undergone degeneration, that are located within the myometrial veins and in distant metastatic sites. The meager response in the former situation is quite different to that observed in a graft reaction, a point that again suggests early choriocarcinoma is a bit at variance with the usual graft phenomena.

Invasion of the stromal core of the villus by its own malignant trophoblast. In one of the two specimens reported here, several stages of this phenomenon were observed. The basement membrane was lost and malignant trophoblastic cells were amidst the stromal cells of the central core. These findings leave no doubt that the malignant trophoblast does invade the stroma of its own villus. However, from our observations this is not a prevalent phenomenon.

A remarkable finding was the failure of the malignant trophoblast to destroy the fetal endothelium of the capillaries which it approximated and its failure to invade the fetal capillaries. Not a single instance of this was observed. This is especially striking in view of the great affinity of trophoblast for maternal blood vessels. This failure may explain why metastatic disease in the fetus is so infrequent.

Loss of the formed villus structure during the developmental stages of choriocarcinoma. In the early stages of development of choriocarcinoma within a normal placenta villi are present, but in the later stages, the ones usually seen by pathologists, villi are absent. This simply means that during the progression of disease the formed villous structure is lost. From the observations of the two specimens reported here it seems possible that the loss can be explained by the prevalent spontaneous regression of the malignant trophoblast and villous core and, to a much lesser extent, by the invasion of the central stromal core by its own trophoblast.

In these two cases villi were absent in the metastatic trophoblastic masses in the veins in the myometrium and in distant metastatic sites, despite the fact that villi accompanied by malignant trophoblast still remained in the primary site. It is apparent that the malignant trophoblast had broken loose from its villous attachment and had been carried by the circulating maternal blood into the maternal vascular system, leaving behind the intact formed villous structure. This phenomenon may occur without associated degenerative changes but in some instances at least, the spontaneous regressive reaction may make it easy for fragments of trophoblastic cell masses to be broken away from its villous attachment.

Summary

Observations have been presented of the characteristic features, previously undescribed, in the early development of choriocarcinoma arising in the placenta of non-molar type.

In these early stages the usual histologic criteria for the diagnosis of choriocarcinoma, namely, absence of villi and hemorrhage into and necrosis of the maternal tissue are all lacking. Despite this, the diagnosis of choriocarcinoma is verified by the fact that the lesion killed both patients and in both the metastatic lesions were typical of choriocarcinoma.

References

DRISCOLL, S. G., Choriocarcinoma: an "incidental finding" within a term placenta. *Obstet. and Gynec.* 21, 96—101 (1963).

McKELVEY, J. L., Personal Communication.

A Study of Choriocarcinoma
Its Incidence in India and Its Aetiopathogenesis

Dr. K. Narayana Pai

B. A., M. B. B. S., D. T. M. H., M. R. C. P. (Edin.)
Professor of Medicine, Medical College and Physician, Medical College Hospital
Trivandrum

The data on the incidence of chorio-carcinoma and vesicular [hydatidiform.- Ed] mole (Table I) were obtained, where available, from the various teaching hospitals of India. The lowest incidence is

Table I. *Incidence of trophoblastic neoplasia in teaching hospitals of India*

Area	Incidence per pregnancy	
	Chorio-carcinoma	Vesicular mole
Trivandrum	1 : 525	1 : 160
Madurai	1 : 1,141	1 : 196
Vellore	1 : 1,857	
Calcutta	1 : 4,000	1 : 400
Madras	1 : 2,958	1 : 361

found in the north of India (Calcutta), increasing as one proceeds south to the highest incidence in the southern most State of Kerala (Trivandrum).

In the Collegiate Women and Children's Hospital in Trivandrum a total of 142 cases of choriocarcinoma have been seen during the past 9 years and 9 months (from Jan. 1955 to Sept. 1964). The total number of obstetric admissions during the same period was 74,509 making an incidence of 1 : 525 pregnancies. The diagnosis of choriocarcinoma was made on

clinical grounds and confirmed by histological examination.

The relative incidence of choriocarcinoma among members of various religious communities is shown in Table II. The

Table II. *Choriocarcinoma among religious communities in Kerala State, India*

Community	No.	%	Incidence of chorio-carcinoma %
Total population	16,903,715		
Hindus	10,300,000	60	59.3
Christians	3,600,000	21.3	32
Muslims	3,000,000	17.9	8
Unknown	3,715	0.8	0.7

high incidence among Christians may be related to the high parity amongst them compared to the other communities.

The relation of the incidence of choriocarcinoma to parity is shown in Table III. Only 35 % occurred in the first 3 pregnancies. Para VI and above constituted only 25 % of all deliveries but nearly half of all cases of choriocarcinoma occurred in this group of patients. Indeed one-fourth occurred after 9 or more pregnancies. Table IV shows that about one-third of total deliveries occurred in women age 30 and more that the incidence of choriocarcinoma was nearly 60% in the same

16 cases it ranged from 1 to 13 years, in 2 of them the onset was 5 years after menopause and 10—13 years after last childbirth.

Table III. *Distribution of choriocarcinoma cases according to parity (percentage)*

Parity	Chorio-carcinoma	Births in Trivandrum city	
I	11.6	22.6	
II	14.0	16.3	Para I—III 52.3%
III	9.3	13.4	
IV	7.0	12.6	Para IV—V 23.5%
V	9.3	10.9	
VI	9.3	8.5	
VII	11.6	6.3	
VIIII	2.3	4.3	Para VI+ 24.2%
IX	7.0	2.4	
X and above	18.6	2.7	
Total	100.0	100.0	

Table IV. *Distribution of choriocarcinoma according to age (in percent)*

Age groups (years)	Chorio-carcinoma %	Births in Trivandrum city	Average number of children
15—19	1.6	9.1	1.2
20—24	40.1	28.4	2.2
25—29		29.6	3.7
30—34	32.0	19.1	5.3
35—39		11.2	6.9
40 and above	26.3	2.6	8.0
		100.0	

group of patients, which also has a lower birth rate but a higher order of parity. This suggests that the incidence of choriocarcinoma rises with the age and parity.

A history of preceding mole was obtained in 55%, abortion in 25% and normal pregnancy in 19%. The interval between the last pregnancy and the onset of symptoms varied from 2 weeks to one year in the majority of the patients. In

Pulmonary metastasis in choriocarcinoma patients were detected in 11 out of 40 cases examined in detail. Other metastases detected were 10 in vulva and vagina, 3 periurethral, 2 in the skin and 1 in the liver.

Treatment

Panhysterectomy and salpingo-oophorectomy were done in the majority of cases.

Until a year or two ago the adjuvant line of treatment consisted mainly of irradiation after hysterectomy. In our country small quantities of methotrexate, cyclophosphamide and vinblastine have become available only in the past two or three years to a few centers for restricted trials.

The survival rate of choriocarcinoma patients in the prechemotherapeutic era was 26 per cent in Trivandrum and 40.75 per cent in Madras. The results with chemotherapy in India are shown in Table V. Though the number of cases treated with methotrexate is small, the results have been similar to those obtained by Manahan, Hertz and Hreshchyshyn and it is now considered the drug of choice in the treatment of choriocarcinoma.

No spontaneous regression of choriocarcinoma occurred in our series and none in the series of Rao from Madras.

especially if they terminate in the early months as abortion or as mole, (2) malnutrition, especially of protein and (3) the presence of active or treated pulmonary tuberculosis. The incidence of pulmonary tuberculosis is high in India but no definite relation of choriocarcinoma to pulmonary tuberculosis could be found. Routine examination of patients with molar pregnancy and skiagram of chest in all cases of suspected choriocarcinoma have failed to reveal pulmonary tuberculosis in our series. Rao from Madras found only one case of pulmonary tuberculosis among 27 patients with choriocarcinoma and 232 cases of hydatidiform mole.

Table V. *Drug therapy of choriocarcinoma in teaching hospitals of India*

Area	Methotrexate		Cyclo-phosphamide		Vinblastine	
	No.	Cured*	No.	Cured	No.	Cured
Trivandrum	3	2	1	1	—	—
Lucknow	—	—	1	0	—	—
Vellore	1	1				
Madurai	7	3				
Calcutta	2	0				
Madras	4	4**			1	0

* Cured: Survival of 1 year or more.
** Hysterectomy + Cobalt beam + Methotrexate — survival 1–6

Discussion

Choriocarcinoma is a common malignant disorder of the southern parts of India. The reasons for this great incidence are not understood. Acosta-Sison has said that in the Philippines the predisposing factors may be (1) frequent pregnancies rapidly succeeding one another

Nutritional factors, especially protein deficiency may play a role in the aetiopathogenesis of choriocarcinoma. The incidence of nutritional disorders is high in Kerala. Beside protein deficiency, folic acid deficiency may also play some as yet unknown part in the maldevelopment of trophoblastic tissues. An analogy may be drawn from the influence of nutritional factors in the etiology of primary carcinoma associated with cirrhosis of the liver, a condition which is very common in Kerala.

The reported high incidence of chorio-carcinoma in older patients with higher parity has been confirmed in our series. Furthermore, the marital fertility rate of 264.9 in Kerala is strikingly high. The economic backwardness, the high birth rate and the high fertility rate in Kerala may be as important contributions to etiologic factors as nutritional deficiencies.

Natural radiation from the thorium rich sands extending for about 150 miles along the west coast of Kerala over an area of half mile wide may have a bearing on carcinogenesis in general. The extent of radiation in this area has been found to be much higher than the maximum permissible World Health Organization standards. Epidemiologic survey and experimental work may help in elucidating any relationship between the high radioactivitiy and high incidence of choriocarcinoma in this part of India.

Observation on Some Aspects of Hydatidiform Mole and Choriocarcinoma in Indonesia

Ariawan Soejoenoes, M. D., Moeljono Djojopranoto, M. D., and Han Tjwan Poen, M. D.

Department of Pathology, School of Medicine, University of Airlangga, Surabaja, Indonesia

Previous publications of several authors from Indonesia leave no doubt as to the high incidence of hydatidiform mole and choriocarcinoma in this country. Although this high incidence of trophoblastic disease is shared by many Asian countries, additional data from Surabaja, Indonesia may contribute to present day knowledge.

The data presented in this paper include patients with hydatidiform mole and choriocarcinoma seen at the General Hospital (Dr. Soetomo Hospital) and the Roman Catholic Hospital. Dr. Soetomo Hospital is a charity hospital, serving a section of the population characterized by low economic and poor nutritional status. The Roman Catholic Hospital is a private hospital serving a small group of the population with a high standard of living and good nutritional habits comparable with western living standards. In Dr. Soetomo Hospital 211 patients with mole were treated during a 5 year period (1960—1964). Five cases of hydatidiform mole occurred in the Roman Catholic Hospital in a 2 year period (1962—1963). The majority of patients with hydatidiform mole (54.1 %) were between 20 and 29 years old which was also true for normal deliveries (54.9 %); the average age was 30 years old for both groups. Above the age of 35 however, there is a relative increase in the incidence of hydatidiform mole. Half the moles occurred in the 1st, 2nd or 3rd pregnancies, whereas the other half occurred among the higher pregnancies which made up only about 40 % of the births. Thus there was a relative increase in incidence with increasing parity.

Bleeding was the main symptom in 97.6 % of patients. One patient died of massive blood loss. Uterine cramps and pain occurred in 53 % of patients, hyperemesis in 19.4 %, and toxemia in 26 % of all cases. One patient convulsed.

Uterine enlargement larger than corresponding gestation was found in 49.8 % of cases.

In considering etiologic factors, the incidence of hydatidiform mole in the Dr. Soetomo and Roman Catholic Hospitals was compared. The respective ratio of hydatidiform mole to the total number of gestations for the two hospitals was 1:85 and 1:373.

It is therefore suggested that lower social conditions especially undernutrition and chronic disease might play an important role in the causation of this disease. Characteristics like age and parity can also be considered as additional influencing factors.

Synopsis of discussion II

Dr. HENDRICKSE reported his experience with the epidemiology of malignant trophoblastic disease in Nigeria since 1954. He has seen 104 cases of whom 60 % were less than 30 years of age. All but 10 of these patients came from within a radius of 100 miles of Ibadan. All but 8 on appearance had metastases. 40 % were primigravida.

Dr. LI speculated that since no American-born Chinese had suffered trophoblastic neoplasia in a survey he had made among the sizable Chinese community in the United States, that heredity, multiparity and late age of pregnancy all seem to be less important than socio-economic or dietary factors in causation of trophoblastic neoplasia. Dr. HSU observed that in Hawaii, where rice is widely eaten, no exceptional incidence of trophoblastic neoplasia was seen comparable to that in Asia. He alluded to studies of a penicillium species which grew on rice and experimentally could induce increased trophoblastic activity as well as other evidences of toxicologic effects. It was moot whether such a contaminant was a factor in human epidemiology. Dr. BURCHENAL remarked that aflatoxin on contaminated food stuffs could induce hepatic tumors experimentally. Dr. KOSS recommended that the International Union undertake a new and intensive study of the epidemiology of trophoblastic neoplasia.

Three examples were cited of multiple moles in succession. Dr. CHUN reported that 5 of 269 patients she had studied had a second mole. Dr. PARK cited epidemiologic information for the British Isles where there are about 13 fatal choriocarcinomas per year. This calculates to approximately one in 50,000 births. The frequency of mole is 1 in 2,000 births.

The malignant transformation of trophoblast in the lung was doubted by Dr. BAGSHAWE who proposed residual persistent trophoblast in the pelvic veins as an alternative, with later embolization. Only 4 of 58 of his patients have shown no evidence of pulmonary embolization during treatment. Dr. CHAN rejoined that 3 of his patients had had hysterectomies one to three years before the presumed emergence of trophoblastic neoplasia in the lungs from transformation in situ. Dr. KOSS cautioned that in human cancer long latent periods before evidence of clinical manifestation were not exceptional and that malignant change in the lung was unlikely.

The Mechanism of Action of Folic Acid Antagonists

James F. Holland, M. D.

Department of Medicine A, Roswell Park Memorial Institute Buffalo 3, New York

The folic acid antagonists enjoy a unique place in cancer chemotherapy (Holland, 1961). Aminopterin was the first designed antimetabolite which provided significant regression of a neoplasm, acute lymphocytic leukemia in children (Farber *et al.*, 1948). Nearly ten years ago, in October 1955, methotrexate was first demonstrated to possess activity which has subsequently proved curative in a majority of trophoblastic neoplasms (Li *et al.*, 1956).

That a single class of antimetabolites can so drastically alter two diseases implies that common targets may be susceptible. It thus is of interest to learn the mechanism of action of these drugs and how they deliver their lethal injury to susceptible cells. The mechanism of natural and of acquired resistance to their action

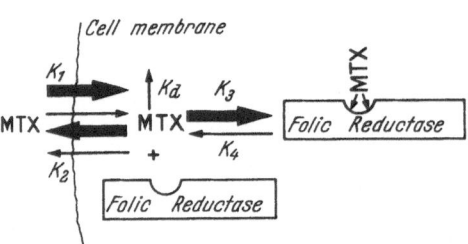

Fig. 1. Schematic activity of methotrexate
(see text)

is also of importance, and leads to consideration of lines of current research which may enhance therapy.

To exhibit its activity, methotrexate must gain entry to the cell, a process in which there is but little competition with folic acid (Fig. 1). Influx of methotrexate to the cell in several cultured lines has been found to be due to passive diffusion rather than active transport (Hakala, 1965). Because methotrexate is a nega-

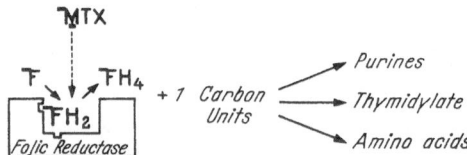

Fig. 2. Schematic role of folic reductase and how methotrexate might serve as a powerful inhibitor

tively charged hydrophilic compound approaching a lipid rich negatively charged cell membrane, permeation of these cells is slow (small arrow). In murine and human leukemic cells, however, active energy-dependent transport and rapid entry has been described (K_1) (Fischer, 1962). Fischer has found varying efficiencies of active transport systems for methotrexate into leukemic leukocytes from different patients. No information is available with respect to trophoblastic tissues.

Once in the cell methotrexate can undergo three fates. Drug destruction has not been persuasively demonstrated (K_d).

Loss of drug from the cell may be a rapid active energy-dependent transfer process such as occurs in cultured sarcoma 180 cells with a rate greater than that of drug tino, 1963). The vast bulk of the drug entering the cell, however, is quickly bound in nearly stoichiometric fashion to folic reductase (K_3).

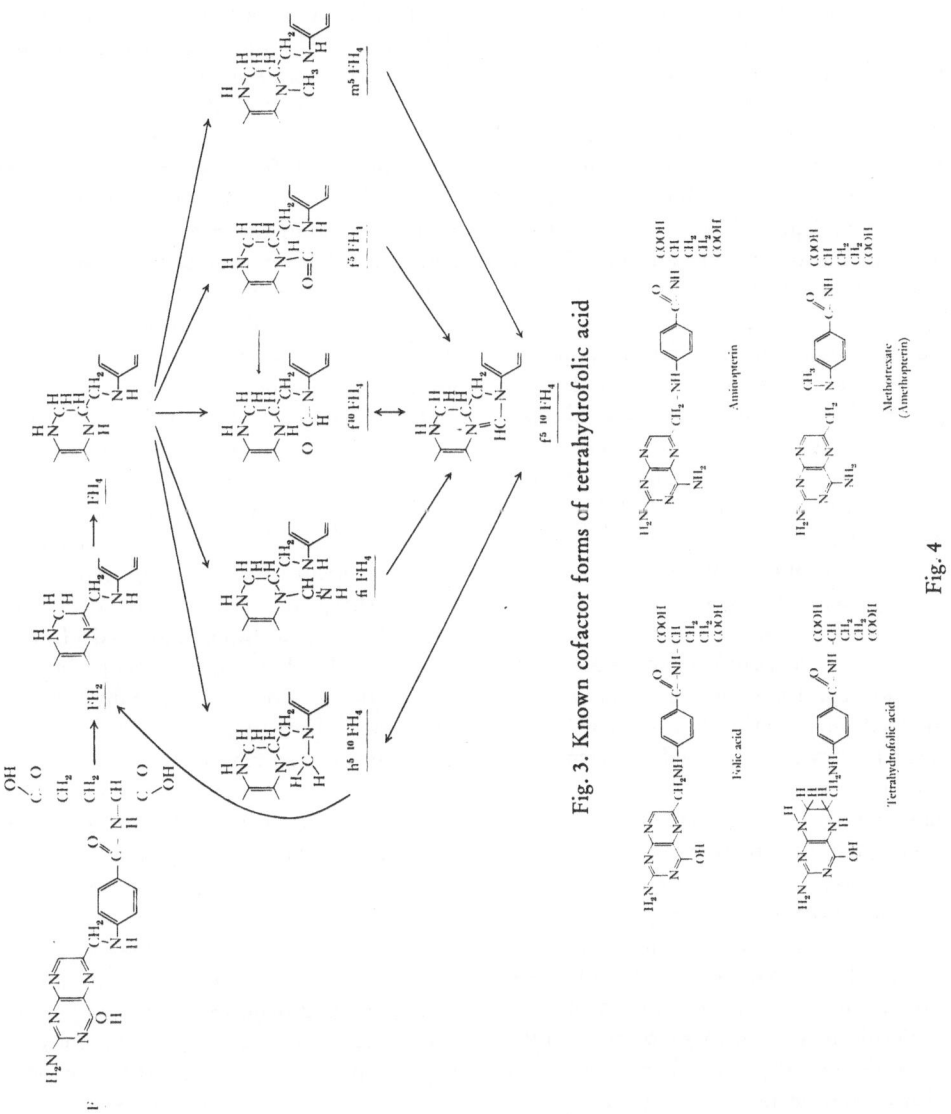

Fig. 3. Known cofactor forms of tetrahydrofolic acid

Fig. 4

entry (HAKALA, 1965), or by passive transfer (K_2). FISCHER has shown differing ability of human leukemic cells to retain methotrexate when placed in a medium free of the drug (FISCHER, quoted in Bertino, ...).

Folic reductase is a nearly ubiquitous enzyme in growing cells (Fig. 2) which serves as the catalyst for reducing folic acid and dihydrofolic acid to tetrahydrofolic acid. Tetrahydrofolate is the active vitamin form. Single carbon compounds at various levels of oxidation are added to tetrahydrofolate and they then are shuttled to metabolic pathways: in the synthesis of thymidylate among the pyrimidines, inosinate among the purines, and amino acid metabolism. The known cofactor forms of tetrahydrofolic acid are shown in Fig. 3. It will be noted in Fig. 4 that an amino group has been substituted for the 4-hydroxyl group of folic acid to make aminopterin which is further altered by a methyl group on the 10-nitrogen to make methotrexate. The additional amino group provides for markedly enhanced hydrogen bonding or electrostatic attraction in the active site of folic reductase. When the active site is thus tenaciously occupied by the antimetabolite, the provitamin folic acid is denied access, tetrahydrofolic acid production is interrupted and the cell is obliged to fulfill its tetrahydrofolic cofactor requirements from existing supplies. Although it has now been persuasively demonstrated that methotrexate can be a competitive inhibitor in vitro for dihydrofolic acid (WANG and WERKEISER, 1964), under in vivo conditions, the drug is tightly if not irreversibly bound (WERKHEISER, 1965). Pharmacologic doses of dihydrofolic acid in man have been found to displace 13% of retained tritiated methotrexate, indicating at least something less than stoichiometric binding (JOHNS et al., 1964).

Since two hydrogen molecules from 5 — 10 - hydroxymethyl - tetrahydrofolate are taken from the tetrahydrofolic acid molecule in the synthesis of thymidylate from deoxyuridylate, this particular synthetic step leads to the production of dihydrofolic acid (Fig. 3). When the active site of folic reductase is blocked by the folic antagonist, the dihydrofolic acid cannot further be reduced to the active tetrahydrofolate form, and cells synthesizing thymidylate at a rapid rate soon

experience intracellular tetrahydrofolate depletion (WERKHEISER, 1961; 1963).

The fourth fate of folic reductase-bound drug is dissociation and liberation back into the intracellular media where it again may undergo any of the first three fates. The dissociation constant of the folic reductase methotrexate is probably of the order of 10^{-11} M (WANG and WERKHEISER, 1964). In vivo, enormous levels of folic reductase have not been found. Although this small dissociation constant in the presence of extreme elevation of folic reductase would allow some free enzyme to satisfy cellular need, it is unlikely that dissociation is a mechanism for resistance in diseases encountered in man. The phenomenon has been recognized, however, as the cause of resistance of highly resistant cells in culture (HAKALA, 1965).

In man, the best concept of the mechanism of action of methotrexate relates to ability to saturate all the folic reductase, and to keep it saturated for sufficient time that intracellular tetrahydrofolate deficiency develops. In some cells, notably liver, storage forms of tetrahydrofolic acid exist which bypass the blockade. In most rapidly growing cells, however, the deficiency may produce lethal injury to the cell because of interruption of vital reactions dependent on tetrahydrofolate cofactors. Resistance represents failure to accomplish this tetrahydrofolic deficiency. Resistance may relate to ineffective penetration of drug to the cell (perhaps due to active cellular drug excretion) with failure to saturate that amount of enzyme present, or to adaptive synthesis of new folic reductase after initial exposure to the drug. BERTINO has demonstrated rise in the folic reductase content of leukemic leukocytes within two days even as the leukocyte concentration in peripheral blood was decreasing (BERTINO, 1963). It is not certain, however, that this is adaptive synthesis of new enzyme. It might be folic reductase which could have been synthesized anyhow, plus that which ordinarily would have disappeared in rapid protein turnover, but is protected from catabolism by being bound to the drug (BERTINO, 1965).

The inhibition of thymidylate and purine biosynthesis by methotrexate is substantially greater than that of protein biosynthesis, and megaloblastosis indicative of disproportionate continuing cytoplasmic protein synthesis is well known (THIERSCH and PHILIPS, 1949). Thus as with other proteins, folic reductase may be synthesized despite the presence of methotrexate. If free methotrexate is available intracellularly, the newly synthesized enzyme is tightly bound and no folic reductase function will be apparent. If, however, the intracellular free drug concentration has become sufficiently low that it does not saturate the newly synthesized folic reductase, the protein may be available for enzymatic function and cellular survival ensue. A slow rate of methotrexate entry would lead to low intracellular drug concentrations and a short time span before folic reductase could exist uninhibited, with refractoriness of that tissue to drug. A fast rate of drug entry, however, would have the opposite effects with high intracellular concentrations, prolonged availability of drug to inhibit folic reductase, and cell sensitivity (WERKHEISER, 1963). In those tissues where folic reductase adaptive synthesis had occurred the additional need for greater intracellular drug concentration would exist.

Although methotrexate effects have been recognized in many reactions using tetrahydrofolic cofactors, none are so exquisitely sensitive as is the effect on folic reductase.

WERKHEISER has postulated that the apparent competitive relationship between methotrexate and citrovorum factor is not indicative of methotrexate activity on a distal enzyme site but rather of a relatively constant ratio of tetrahydrofolic acid compounds and methotrexate in tissues. Higher intracellular concentrations of free methotrexate (which last longer) would take higher intracellular amounts of citrovorum factor to protect the cell against critical tetrahydrofolate deficiency, until methotrexate concentration reached zero and new folic reductase synthesis was able to provide for tetrahydrofolate requirements (WERKHEISER, 1965).

Since the essence of all chemotherapy is selective toxicity, in which the host sustains less injury than the tumor, all the foregoing considerations must be acomplished under conditions which leave vital systems of the host sublethally intoxicated. In some instances the host's integrity is maintained, not apparently by lesser toxicity, but by more rapid regeneration of injured tissue.

What are the relations of these observations to natural sensitivity and resistance? The Walker 256 carcinoma of rats is highly refractory to methotrexate administration (ROSEN and NICHOL, 1962) whereas the Murphy-Sturm lymphosarcoma is highly susceptible. WERKHEISER transplanted one of each tumor type into the same rat, administered varying doses of methotrexate, and measured folic reductase inhibition in each tumor and in gut mucosa, the toxicologically most vulnerable tissue. He found that the median lethal dose was almost precisely the dose necessary to reduce free folic reductase of intestinal mucosa to negligible levels, thus impeding synthesis of essential compounds for replacement of the rapidly growing gut epithelium. The folic reductase of the sensitive Murphy-Sturm lymphosarcoma was completely inhibited at dose levels lower than those required to inhibit the folic reductase of the gut mucosa, whereas that of Walker carcinoma 256 was not completely inhibited, even at doses of the drug which quantitatively inhibited the gut enzyme and were associated with death of more than half of the animals. Thus success in treating the lymphosarcoma is ascribable to a greater drug effectiveness on tumor enzyme than on the most sensitive host tissue folic reductase. The refractoriness of Walker carcinoma would not appear to be absolute. Indeed folic reductase of that tumor was inhibited by methotrexate but at a rate less than that of gut mucosa. Thus, toxic and lethal effects on the host occurred before complete inhibition of the target enzyme in refractory tumor (WERKHEISER, 1963). Permeability to drug of mouse leukemic cells as compared to gut also seemed to be the critical variable in determining sensitivity (WERKHEISER et al., 1963).

The difference in permeability for folic antagonists can also be seen for folic acid in deficient diets. Thus Walker carcinoma 256 which has a low uptake of folic antagonists and is refractory to drug, is highly susceptible to folic acid deprivation in the diet (ROSEN and NICHOL, 1962). Contrariwise, Murphy-Sturm lymphosarcoma, highly susceptible to methotrexate, also concentrates folic acid and is refractory to dietary deficiency (WERKHEISER, 1963).

Relative causes for refractoriness to methotrexate in the natural state or induced by prior exposure to the drug may include, in addition to factors already considered, failure to deliver the drug to the tumor, and the capacity of neoplastic tissue to utilize alternative preformed substrates such as purines, pyrimidines and serum 5-methyltetrahydrofolate (HERBERT et al., 1962). Host intolerance to the drug may be conditioned by dietary folic deficiency or induced deficiency from a rapidly proliferating tumor or hematopoietic tissue using up folate acti-vity, principally 5-methyltetrahydrofolate from serum and hepatic stores.

Exaggerated serum concentrations of methotrexate from poor renal excretion often accounts for therapeutic failure from excessive toxicity and can usually be anticipated by elevation of the serum creatinine or blood urea nitrogen concentration.

The two major considerations that emerge as bases for success or failure of tumor chemotherapy vis a vis toxicity for the host are attainment and maintenance of high intracellular methotrexate concentrations and the adaptive synthesis of folic reductase. Permeability characteristics of folic antagonists are now receiving attention of organic chemists, and the highly polar group in the glutamate moiety may soon be substituted or eliminated completely. WERKHEISER (1965) found that elimination probably would not seriously affect enzyme binding yet might enhance drug entry to cell.

Secondly, the appearance of folic reductase as a mechanism of resistance has been turned into a therapeutic weapon. A search has been made by Friedkin and his colleagues for compounds that might be inactive in the oxidized form, but when reduced by folic reductase exhibit inhibitory activity on thymidylic synthetase (FRIEDKIN, 1963). GOODMAN et al., (1964) have recently synthesized homofolic acid which is chemically reducible to dihydrohomofolic acid. Dihydrohomofolate is reduced by folic reductase as well as is dihydrofolate. The product, tetrahydrohomofolate (same structure as tetrahydrofolate in Figure 4 except for one additional methylene group between tetrahydropteridine and para aminobenzoate moieties) is a powerful inhibitor of thymidylate synthetase. No animal chemotherapeutic studies are yet reported for this compound, but the use of the biochemical rationale, a lethal synthesis by the cells with acquired resistance, and preliminary activity data for *Streptococ-* *cus faecalis* and *Lactobacillus casei* are encouraging.

References

BERTINO, J. R. The mechanism of action of the folate antagonists in man. *Cancer Res.* 23, 1286—1306 (1963).
— Current studies of the folate antagonists in patients with acute leukemia. *Cancer Res.* 25, 1614—1619 (1965).
FARBER, S., DIAMOND, L. K., MERCER, R. D., SYLVESTER, R. F., JR., and WOLFF, J. A., Tempory remissions in acute leukemia in children produced by folic acid antagonists, 4-aminopteroylglutamic acid (aminopterin). *New Engl. J. Med.* 238, 787—793 (1948).
FISCHER, G. A., Cited in Bertino, *Cancer Res.*
— Defective transport of amethopterin (methotrexate) as a mechanism of resistance of the antimetabolite in L5178Y leukemic cells. *Biochem. Pharmacol.* 11, 1233—1234 (1962).
FRIEDKIN, M., Cited in Nichol, C. A., Summary of informal discussions on the role of folic acid antagonists. *Cancer Res.* 23, 1307 (1963).
GOODMAN, L., DeGRAW, J., KISLIUK, R. L., FRIEDKIN, M., PASTORE, E. J., CRAWFORD, E. J., PLANTE, L. T., AL-HAHAS, A., MORNINGSTAR, J. F., JR., KWOK, G., WILSON, L., DONOVAN, E. F., and RATZAN, J., Tetrahydrohomofolate, a specific inhibitor of thymidylate synthetase. *J. Amer. chem. Soc.* 86, 308 (1964).
HAKALA, M. T., On the role drug penetration in amethopterin resistance of sarcoma 180 cells *in vitro. Biochim. biophys. Acta (Amst.)* 102, 198—209 (1965).
— On the nature of permeability of sarcoma 180 cells to amethopterin *in vitro. Biochim. biophys. Acta (Amst.)* 102, 210—225 (1965).
HERBERT, V., LARRABEE, A. R., and BUCHANAN, J. M., Studies on the identification of a folate compound of human serum. *J. clin. Invest.* 41, 1134—1138 (1962).
HOLLAND, J. F., Symposium: antimetabolites. Part VII. Folic acid antagonists. *Clin. Pharmacol. Ther.* 2, 374—409 (1961).
JOHNS, D. G., HOLLINGSWORTH, J. W., CASHMORE, A. R., PLENDERLEITH, and BERTINO, J. R., Methotrexate displacement in man. *J. clin. Invest.* 43, 621—629 (1964).
LI, M. C., HERTZ, R., and SPENCER, D. B., Effect of methotrexate therapy upon choriocarcinoma and chorioadenoma. *Proc. Soc. exp. Biol. (N.Y.)* 93, 361—366 (1956).
ROSEN, F., and NICHOL, C. A., Inhibition of the growth of an amethopterin refractory tumor by dietary restriction of folic acid. *Cancer Res.* 22, 495—500 (1962).
THIERSCH, J. B., and PHILIPS, F. S. Effects of 4-aminopteroylglutamic acid in dogs with special reference to megaloblastosis. *Proc. Soc. exp. Biol. (N. Y.)* 71, 484—490 (1949).
WANG, D. H., and WERKHEISER, W. C., Mechanism of inhibition of folate reductase (FR) by 4-amino folate antagonists. *Fed. Proc.* 23, 324 (1964).
WERKHEISER, W. C., Specific binding of 4-amino folic acid analogues by folic acid reductase. *J. biol. Chem.* 236, 888—893 (1961).
— The biochemical, cellular and pharmacological action and effects of the folic acid antagonists. *Cancer Res.* 23, 1277—1285 (1963).
— Limitations on the therapeutic effectiveness of the folic acid antagonists. *Cancer Res.* 25, 1608—1613 (1965).
— LAW, L., ROOSA, R. A., and NICHOL, C. A., Further evidence that selective uptake modifies cellular response to the 4-amino folate antagonists. *Proc. Amer. Ass. Cancer Res.* 4, 71 (1963).

Eight Years Experience with the Chemotherapy of Choriocarcinoma and Related Trophoblastic Tumors in Women

Roy Hertz, M. D., Ph. D.

Endocrinology Branch, National Cancer Institute, Bethesda, Maryland

This report briefly summarizes our experience with the chemotherapy of choriocarcinoma and related trophoblastic tumors in women during the eight years since the initial report by Li, Hertz and Spencer (1956). The data to be presented are derived from 116 cases with metastases and 38 cases with disease presumably confined to the uterus.

Analysis of these cases has revealed numerous features of the natural history of trophoblastic pathology in women. This has led us to the concept that the clinical entities of hydatidiform mole, chorioadenoma destruens [invasive mole-Ed.]), and choriocarcinoma actually constitute a spectrum of abnormalities of the chorion rather than distinctly separable categories of disease. This view stems from the fact that normal chorionic tissue represents the common antecedent structure from which all of these tumor processes are derived. Moreover, it is well documented that about one half of patients presenting with choriocarcinoma have an antecedent history of hydatidiform mole. In addition, among 39 autopsies we have found only two instances of persistent villous structures although 15 of these patients had previously exhibited a molar pregnancy. In numerous instances we have adequate microscopic material from both biopsy and autopsy material clearly reflecting the progression of the disease process.

Accordingly, we have employed the term "trophoblastic disease" to designate those pathological states associated with the morphological finding of hydatidiform mole, chorioadenoma destruens or choriocarcinoma as defined by Novak and Seah (1954). The term "metastatic trophoblastic disease" is applied to those cases in which the tumor process has extended beyond the uterus. In addition, the histopathological diagnosis as revealed in tissues available at the time of admission is noted for each case.

Our diagnostic and therapeutic criteria as well as our methods of observation, treatment and evaluation have been fully described in previous reports and will not be detailed here (Hertz et al., 1958; Hertz et al., 1961; Ross et al., 1965; Ross et al., 1962).

Our entire chemotherapeutic experience with metastatic trophoblastic disease is tabulated in Table I. This group of 121 cases is subdivided into: Series "A" consisting of 63 cases treated mainly with methotrexate until either remission or refractoriness ensued. In the latter instance vinblastine and in a few scattered cases other oncolytic agents were applied. Series "B" consists of 50 cases seen subsequently who were treated by the successive application of methotrexate and actinomycin D or conversely by actinomycin D followed by methotrexate.

Series "C" consists of a group of 13 patients who were referred to us after various ineffectual regimens of chemotherapy and were subsequently treated by us with

37, or 74 % have experienced complete remission.

It is noteworthy that the effectiveness of these agents when applied alone or suc-

Table I. *Results of treatment in 116 cases of metastatic trophoblastic disease*

Series	Chemo-therapy prior to admission	No. of patients	Histopathology complete remissions/total	
			Chorio	Mole, destruens and others
A MTX, VLB 1956—1961	none	63	21/44 (48 %)	9/19 (47 %)
B** MTX, Actino 1961—1964	none	50	22/29 (76 %)	15/21 (71 %)
C MTX, Actino, Combs. 1961—1964	varied regimens *	13	1/10 (10 %)	3/3 (100 %)

* Includes MTX, Actino, HN_2, VLB.
** Includes 5 cases alive with disease from Series A.

a variety of oncolytic agents either singly or in combination. Because of the complicating feature of prior treatment by other regimens the 13 cases in Series "C" are not included in our evaluation of the effectiveness of our own therapeutic procedures. It will be noted that Table I also divides our cases as to histopathological diagnosis on admission.

Without undue detail, it may be stated that about half of our patients with metastatic trophoblastic disease have experienced a complete and sustained remission following either methotrexate alone or actinomycin D alone. Of the remaining patients who develop resistance to either agent, about half can be brought into complete remission by secondary application of the agent not previously applied, whether this be methotrexate or actinomycin D (Table II). Thus in the last 50 cases of Series "B" treated by the sequential application of these two agents

cessively in patients with metastases is not materially affected by the ante-mortem histological diagnosis. This suggests that

Table II. *Response to chemotherapy in 50 patients with metastatic trophoblastic disease.*

Regimen	Total patients	Remission
MTX alone or followed by actinomycin D *	36	26 (72 %)
Actinomycin D alone or followed by MTX *	14	11 (79 %)
Totals	50	37 (74 %)

* In resistant cases.

factors of host-tumor relationship other than those reflected in morphology play a vital role in the outcome of metastatic trophoblastic disease (Table III).

Table III. *Influence of duration of disease, histological diagnosis, and initial gonadotropin titer on response to chemotherapy in last 50 cases*

Duration of disease (months)	Complete remissions/total patients						
	Titer $<1\times10^6$ M. U.			Titer $>1\times10^6$ M. U.			
	Chorioca	Other*	All histological types	Chorioca	Other	All histological types	Totals
4 or less	11/12	9/9	20/21 (95%)	2/2	1/4	3/6 (50%)	23/27 ** (85%)
Over 4	6/7	4/5	10/12 (84%)	3/8	1/3	4/11 (36%)	14/23 ** (61%)
Both time groups combined	17/19	13/14	30/33 *** (91%)	5/10	2/7	7/17 *** (41%)	37/50 (74%)

  * Hydatidiform mole, chorioadenoma destruens, syncitial endometritis, and other tissue diagnoses.
  ** p = <0.025
  *** p = <0.001

The great importance of such factors of interaction between tumor and host is reflected in the critical role which the

Table IV. *Influence of duration of disease on outcome*

Duration of disease (in months)	Complete remissions (total patients)	
	Series A	Series B
4 or less	18/25 (72%)	23/27 (85%)
4 or more	12/38 (31%)	14/23 (61%)
Totals	30/63 (48%)	37/50 (74%)

prior duration of disease plays in the ultimate response to chemotherapy (Table III and IV). If this factor alone is considered we observe that among 23 of our most recent 50 patients in whom chemotherapy was initiated after 4 months of illness only a 61% complete remission rate is obtained, whereas among 27 patients treated before 4 months of illness an 85% remission rate is seen. The importance of this time factor is comparable for all histological types. The importance

of this factor was similarly observed in our earlier series of 63 cases (Hertz, et. al. 1958).

Table V. *Effect of initial titer on response to chemotherapy*

Titer (m. u. u./24 hrs)	Complete remissions (total patients)	
	Series A	Series B
Up to 1 million	19/32 (56%)	30/33 (91%)
1 million and over	11/31 (34%)	7/17 (41%)
Totals	30/63 (48%)	37/50 (74%)

Moreover, if one considers the gonadotropin titer encountered just prior to the initiation of chemotherapy in our last 50 cases we observe that an initial urinary excretion titer of less than 1,000,000 mouse uterine units per 24 hours is associated with a 91% remission rate, but only a 41% remission rate is seen in those cases with a greater titer. Also in our earlier series of 63 cases titers of less than 1 million mouse uterine units were associated with remissions in 56 % of 32 cases whereas only 34 % of 31 cases with greater titers experienced complete remission (Table III and V).

Hence our entire experience would serve to emphasize the critical necessity for early diagnosis and therapy. It is also pertinent to emphasize the futility of undue delay for numerous successive diag-

Our data further show that prior hysterectomy (Table VI) has no significant effect on chemotherapeutic response in metastatic trophoblastic disease. Moreover, we have observed numerous instances in which rapid dissemination of disease has occurred shortly after pelvic surgery, suggesting that embolization during surgery has predisposed to such spread of

Table VI. *Effect of prior hysterectomy upon chemotherapeutic response*

| Prior hysterectomy | Complete remissions/total patients | | Total cases |
	1961	1964	
Yes	19/41 (47 %)	21/24 (87 %)	40/65 (61 %)
No	11/22 (50 %)	16/26 (61 %)	27/48 (57 %)

Table VII. *Histopathological diagnosis in patients with non-metastatic trophoblastic disease*

| Last pregnancy | No. patients | Histopathologic diagnoses * | | |
		Hydatidiform mole	Consistent with choriocarcinoma	Other
Molar	29	29	3	3
Term	5	—	5	—
Abortal	4	—	2	2

* Made on tissues recovered by dilatation and curettage.

nostic surgical procedures aimed at determining the histological type of trophoblastic disease, since our experience demonstrates this feature to have little bearing upon the ultimate response to chemotherapy.

The significance of the time factor appears to reflect a process of continuous adaptation between host and tumor tissue which ultimately supports the survival of tumor cells in an intially less favorable environment. In addition, tumor progression from less malignant histological types to more malignant phases of trophoblastic disease may be manifested by decreasing chemotherapeutic responsiveness as time elapses.

disease. Accordingly, we now utilize surgical procedures only when they prove necessary for the control of hemorrhage or other local problems.

These considerations together with our increasingly favorable results from chemotherapy in metastatic disease have stimulated our most recent studies on the primary use of chemotherapy instead of surgery in 38 patients with non-metastatic trophoblastic disease (Table VII). These patients include 29 women who had delivered a hydatid mole at least 30 days prior to treatment and had a persistently elevated gonadotropin titer. Nine of these patients had had either a term pregnancy or an abortion. Histological diagnosis

Table VIII. *Interval between delivery and initiation of chemotherapy*

Last pregnancy	No. patients	<2 Months	2—6 Months	>6 Months
Molar	29	7	19	3
Term	5	0	4	1
Abortal	4	1	2	1

from curettements was considered "consistent with choriocarcinoma". Because of the vagaries of histological diagnosis from

to respond completely and is currently on other therapy. Seven of the nine patients with lesions "consistent with choriocarcinoma" experienced complete remissions and two of these patients also went into complete remission following subsequent hysterectomy. Hence in 38 women with non-metastatic disease, hysterectomy was avoided in 35 patients in whom it would have been otherwise indicated. Table X indicates the duration of these remissions and lists the normal pregnancies which

Table IX. *Time and number of courses of drug for remission*

Last pregnancy	No. patients	Interval in days * (Range)	No. of courses MTX (Range)
Molar	28	36 (15—61)	2.5 (1—4)
Term	3	32 (18—48)	2.2 (1—3)
Abortal	4	45 (23—63)	3.6 (2—5)

* Initiation of chemotherapy to remission.

Table X. *Duration of remission* and subsequent pregnancies*

Last pregnancy	No. patients	Duration >1 yr.	Remission >2 yrs.	Subsequent pregnancy
Molar	28	13	15	8
Term	3	1	2	2
Abortal	4	2	2	2

* As of December 10, 1964.

such material we prefer to regard these patients from a clinical point of view as representing cases of peristent, non-metastatic trophoblastic disease. The duration of disease is indicated in Table VIII. The length of treatment and number of courses of methotrexate given are indicated in Table IX. With one exception, all of the post-mole patients experienced a prompt and complete remission. However, one post-mole patient who had had her molar pregnancy one year before therapy failed

have thus far been experienced by these patients.

In evaluating these results in the post-mole cases one should not disregard the known spontaneous clearing of disease in an undetermined percentage of such cases. However, DELFS (1959) and BREWER (1961) report the occurrence of chorioadenoma in about one fifth and of choriocarcinoma in about one-fifth of such patients. Moreover, the regularity of the response and the minimal hazard of irreversible drug toxicity in these non-debilitated patients more than justify immediate chemotherapy in such cases.

The question naturally arises as to the possible role of completely prophylactic chemotherapy to be universally applied in all patients who have had a molar pregnancy. It has been our practice to avoid such routine prophylactic chemotherapy since such treatment can be avoided in most cases by closely monitoring the chorionic gonadotropin titer in the first month or two after evacuation of the uterus. Where adequate hormonal and clinical follow-up may not be readily available, prophylactic chemotherapy may possibly serve a useful purpose.

We have previously discussed the problem of toxicity attributable to the employment of such intensive therapeutic regimens (HERTZ et. al. 1958; HERTZ et. al., 1961; ROSS et. al. 1965; ROSS et. al., 1962). Such undesirable effects are inherent in this form of management. However, our experience indicates that with proper patient selection and with the application of vigorous medical, laboratory, and nursing support such toxic

effects will prove reversible and represent an acceptable clinical risk. However, it should be equally clear that patients in poor clinical and nutritional state or patients with previously impaired hepatic, renal, or bone marrow function require special consideration.

The question is reasonably raised as to the actual necessity for such highly intensive therapy. Since our experience is limited to the application of the regimens we have described, we can not comment definitively on this point. However, our Series "C" (Table I) consists of 13 patients with persistent trophoblastic disease who had received a variety of less intensive regimens elsewhere prior to admission to our service.

Although this represents a selected group of failures, nevertheless this experience together with numerous verbal accounts of unsatisfactory experience with less intensive regimens elsewhere indicates that intensive, intermittent therapy carefully monitored at both a clinical and laboratory level offers the best prospects for complete remissions.

References

BREWER, J. I., 1961 Textbook of Gynecology, ed. 3. Baltimore, Maryland: WILLIAMS & WILKINS CO.

DELFS, E., *In: Trophoblast and Its Tumors*, OBER, W. B., ed. *Ann. N. Y. Acad. Sci.* 80, 125—139 (1959).

HERTZ, R., BERGENSTAL, D. M., LIPSETT, M. B., PRICE, E. B., and HILBISH, T. F., Chemotherapy of choriocarcinoma and related trophoblastic tumors in women. *J. Amer. med. Ass.* 168, 845—854 (1958).

— LEWIS, J., JR., and LIPSETT, M. B., Five years experience with the chemotherapy of metastatic choriocarcinoma and related trophoblastic tumors in women. *Amer. J. Obstet. Gynec.* 82, 631—640 (1961).

LI, M. C., HERTZ, R., and SPENCER, D. B., Effect of methotrexate therapy upon

choriocarcinoma and chorioadenoma. *Proc. Soc. exp. Biol. (N.Y.)* 93, 361—366 (1956).

NOVAK, E., and SEAH, C. S., Choriocarcinoma of uterus: Study of 74 cases from Mathieu Registry. *Amer. J. Obstet. Gynec.* 67, 933—961 (1954).

ROSS, G. T., GOLDSTEIN, D. P., HERTZ, R., LIPSETT, M. B., and ODELL, W., D., Sequential use of methotrexate and Actinomycin D in the treatment of metastatic choriocarcinoma and related trophoblastic disease in women. *Amer. J. Obstet. Gynec.* 93, 223—229 (1965).

— STOLBACH, L. L., and HERTZ, R., Actinomycin D in the treatment of methotrexate-resistant trophoblastic disease in women. *Cancer Res.* 22, 1015—1017 (1962).

On the Prevention and Treatment of Choriocarcinoma

Constantino P. Manahan, M. D., Rainerio Abad, M. D.,
and Anatalia M. Lopez, M. D.

Department of Obstetrics and Gynecology, College of Medicine,
University of the Philippines and the Philippine General Hospital, Manila,
Philippines

In trying to account for the confusion and the many attempts at classifying mole, chorioadenoma destruens and choriocarcinoma, it seemed to us that the difficulty was in considering these entities as three separate and distinct conditions rather than accepting them as stages in the progression from a benign state, hydatidiform mole, to a highly malignant phase, choriocarcinoma. All these stages may be present in one patient at the same time. The histopathologic features of each of these conditions are universally accepted. While these categories differ in pathologic findings and in behavior, they may be better understood if they are pictured as one condition which we prefer to call trophoblastic disease [neoplasia — Ed]. This concept we have been teaching our students for the past twelve years and to us, in the Philippines, where the incidence of chorionic malignancy is high, the danger of progression from a benign mole to choriocarcinoma has always to be kept in mind. We have placed less emphasis on the histologic grading of a mole, for while it is true that a Grade I mole follows a more benign course than moles with greater trophoblastic activity, still moles supposedly Grade I have developed into chorioadenoma destruens or into metastatic choriocarcinoma. It is admitted that these instances may have been due to poor sampling of the molar specimen sent to the laboratory for examination. However, this but serves to emphasize the difficulty in obtaining the proper sample for examination and the pitfalls which may bring about a false sense of security if prognosis and follow up were to depend to a great extent on histological grading. This emphasis on histologic grading is the reason, too, why on curettage on some occasions the report is made of "syncitial endometritis" only to have the patient die of choriocarcinoma a year later.

More importance has been placed on (1) the early diagnosis of mole, (2) a more careful and adequate follow up of the patient, (3) early adequate treatment, and (4) the prophylactic use of methotrexate in one or two courses to the point of toxicity in cases of mole with the hope of destroying residual and potentially malignant trophoblastic tissue.

The early diagnosis and treatment of choriocarcinoma begins with the early diagnosis and adequate treatment of the so-called benign mole.

The unique relationship of the trophoblast to the maternal host permits a gamut of changes from a benign abnormal villus to choriocarcinoma. The unpredictable reactions of the host which may be systemic or local or both may result in the spontaneous "bizarre" regressions of the tumor, or in a dormancy for long periods of time, for months and even years. On the other hand, in most of our cases, the progression from benign mole to metastatic choriocarcinoma is quite rapid.

That the early diagnosis of a mole is a desideratum is demonstrated by the fact that the cure rate of trophoblastic disease is influenced by the duration of the disease whether spread has taken place or not at the time of chemotherapy. Fifty per cent of the highly malignant stage, choriocarcinoma, are said to arise from mole. ACOSTA-SISON (1964) in following up the cases of hydatidiform mole found 17 per cent to develop into trophoblastic malignancy. In reporting our experience with choriocarcinoma in the Philippines, we (MANAHAN et. al., 1964) noted that during the eight years before the availability of methotrexate, 58 cases of choriocarcinoma were treated, mostly by hysterectomy, with a five-year salvage of 27.5 per cent. When the lesion was early and confined to the uterus, the salvage rate was 90 per cent in contrast to a 10 per cent salvage when the lesion was already metastatic. With the employment of methotrexate, the overall cure rate rose from 27 to 64 per cent. Encouraging as were the results with chemotherapy, whether by surgery and methotrexate or with methotrexate alone without resorting to hysterectomy, still the importance of early diagnosis and treatment became evident. When the lesion was early and

confined to the uterus, chemotherapy yielded a hundred per cent cure. Where it was late and metastases had taken place, the cure rate with chemotherapy was only 50 per cent. In general, where the duration of illness was at least six months, the cure rate was only half that of the group in which the lesion was less than six months in duration.

Since our original study of 41 cases of trophoblastic disease with chorioadenoma and choriocarcinoma reported in October 1963, we have collected from five Manila Hospitals 76 additional cases thus bringing the number studied to 117. Seventy-eight out of 117 are alive and well for a 66 per cent salvage. Of special interest were twenty-two young women, eight on curettage had choriocarcinoma supposedly still confined to the uterus and fourteen already had lung lesions. All had a duration of illness of less than six months as dated from the time the mole was diagnosed. Since most were young, nulliparous or Para I's, hysterectomy was not carried out and methotrexate alone was used. In all, after three to six courses of methotrexate, the urine chorionic gonadotropin became negative and the uterine as well as the lung lesions disappeared. Complete regression of the lung lesions required an average of ten weeks. Ten of these patients have, since the treatment, delivered once, and two have had two full-term deliveries each. There were four abortions in the group.

The experience with these 22 patients satisfy us as to the efficacy of chemotherapy when instituted early and the fact that a hysterectomy need not be an integral part of the treatment of trophoblastic neoplasia with or without metastases.

This does not mean that we advocate doing away with surgery in the treatment of choriocarcinoma or chorioadenoma. We previously had reported cases of chorioadenoma destruens [invasive mole — Ed.] where sensitivity to the drug forced us to carry out a pelvic clean up. Even in the young patient with choriocarcinoma or chorioadenoma where the uterus remains large, where the adnexae are indurated and fixed, where especially there is continued bleeding after at least two good courses of methotrexate, or where a sufficient length of time has elapsed but no regression has taken place, an exploratory laparotomy should be carried out with the intent of performing a hysterectomy and bilateral salpingo-oophorectomy. In the patient who is elderly or who has had her share of children, we still feel that a pelvic clean up should be performed *after* one course of chemotherapy. After surgery, she should receive still another course or courses depending on the urine gonadotropin levels and the behaviour of the metastatic lesions if any are present.

How is the diagnosis of mole made? Hydatidiform mole is recognized by the usual accepted methods and by remembering, so as not to overlook it, that hydatidiform moles are seen in 1 out of 200 pregnancies in our ward cases. Since under certain circumstances a mole may be hard to differentiate from a normal intrauterine pregnancy, especially a multiple pregnancy, the immunologic test of Pascasio developed in our Department is noteworthy. The hemagglutination technic of Boyden as modified by Wide and Gemzell was used. For sensitization of 1 volume of formalinized cells, 0.1 ml of diluted molar fluid added to 1 volume of pH 6.4 phosphate buffer was employed. Normal pregnancies gave negative reactions or positive reactions with titers of 1:20 to 1:40. Positive hemagglutinations were noted in the sera of hydatidiform mole cases, the titers varying from 1:40 to 1:2,560. There is suggestive evidence that there are circulating hemag-

glutinating antibodies to molar fluid. The sera, when reacted with cells sensitized to normal placental homgenate or human chorionic gonadotropin, gave titers of 0 to 1:20 with the former and negative reactions with the latter. The finding that significant titers were obtained in the sera of patients with hydatidiform mole, when reacted with formalinized cells sensitized with molar fluid derived from different patients, suggests the presence of a common antigenic determinant. Moreover, the insignificant titers obtained with normal placental antigen and human chorionic gonadotropin indicate that neither of these are responsible for antibody formation. These studies are being continued.

Having made the diagnosis of hydatidiform mole, what is considered adequate treatment? Evacuation of the molar products by curettage or by hysterotomy has been advised depending on the condition of the cervix. In the elderly patient or in the multipara when blood for transfusion is not available, hysterectomy with the mole in situ has been considered adequate treatment. Following this or following evacuation of the uterus, repeated chorionic gonadotropin determination should be performed.

Certain circumstances have made us change our management of patients with hydatidiform moles. At least 50 per cent of cases are lost to follow up. Hysterectomy is not a complete cure as in an occasional patient lung lesions are noticed one or two weeks after hysterectomy. Moreover, this procedure may be carried out only in the elderly patient or in the patient with many children. Recently, we saw a 45-year old patient who two years after the passage of mole developed a suburethral lesion. This host resistance phenomenon which allows a lesion to lie dormant for months and even years and the fact that at least 50 per cent of our cases, in spite of repeated warnings, do not come back for follow up has made it justifiable for us to follow evacuation of the uterus of the molar products with at least one course of intensive methotrexate therapy given to the point of toxicity. At the start we believed we could prevent trophoblastic proliferation with a dose of 75 mgm of methotrexate (MANAHAN et. al., 1961). A subsequent study reported in another hospital in Manila gave glowing reports. However, four of these patients given 75 mgm of methotrexate and lost to follow up were eventually admitted elsewhere with terminal lung lesions. We believe that to do any good the course of methotrexate should be given to the point of toxicity and in the more anaplastic lesions the course should be repeated.

Summary and conclusion

1. Mole, chorioadenoma destruens and choriocarcinoma are but phases of one condition—trophoblastic neoplasia.

2. Since 50 per cent of choriocarcinomas are said to arise from moles and 17 per cent of moles lead to chorionic malignancy, the early and adequate treatment of choriocarcinoma begins with the early diagnosis and adequate treatment of hydatidiform mole.

3. An immunologic test for the early diagnosis of mole is presented.

4. To adequately treat benign mole, especially where follow up of the patient is not always possible, methotrexate in one or two courses to the point of toxicity should follow delivery of the molar products.

References

ACOSTA-SISON, H., Our changed attitude in the management of hydatidiform mole in 196 cases admitted to the Philippine General Hospital from April 10, 1959 to March 27, 1963. *Phil. J. Surg.* 19, 227—231 (1964).

MANAHAN, C. P., BENITEZ, I., and ESTRELLA, F., Amethopterin in the treatment of trophoblastic tumors. *Amer. J. Obstet. Gynec.* 82, 641—645 (1961).

MANAHAN, C. P., MANUEL-LIMSON, G., and ABAD, R., Experience with choriocarcinoma in the Philippines. *Ann. N. Y. Acad. Sci.* 114, 875—880 (1964).

Chemotherapeutic Prophylaxis Against the Development of Choriocarcinoma Following the Removal of Hydatidiform Mole

Kohachiro Koga, M. D., and Kazuo Maeda, M. D.

Department of Obstetrics and Gynecology, Faculty of Medicine, Kyushu University, Fukuoka, Japan

Systemic chemotherapy within 3 weeks after removal of mole was given to 92 patients in an attempt to prevent the development of chorionepithelioma. Fifty-three patients were treated with Amethopterin, usually 10 mg daily for 5—10 days. In 10 of these patients, Amethopterin was also instilled into the uterine cavity along with the systemic therapy. Thirty-nine patients were treated with other drugs: Nitrogen mustard N-oxide, thio-TEPA, Cyclophosphamide, Mitomycin C, and Chromomycin A3. Thirty-seven patients received no chemotherapy and served as a control.

Choriocarinoma developed in 3 (8.1 per cent) in the control group, 3 (7.7 per cent) in patients treated with drugs other than Amethopterin, and in none of the patients who received prophylactic therapy with Amethopterin. In the group receiving Amethopterin, fewer patients had persistent positive Friedman's test of 100 rabbit units or more one month after removal of hydatidiform mole.

Treatment with chemotherapeutic agents after removal of hydatidiform mole is deemed to be useful in prophylaxis of trophoblastic neoplasia.

An Observation on the Prophylactic Use of Chemotherapy After Termination of Hydatidiform Mole

D. Chun, T. Lu, and H. K. Chung

Department of Obstetrics and Gynaecology
University of Hong Kong

The much dreaded complication of hydatidiform mole is choriocarcinoma and its incidence was found to be 9% among 265 cases treated in our clinic (Chun *et al.*, 1964). A study was made 9 months ago to see if the prophylactic use of chemotherapy could prevent it!

Material and Method

In a series of 14 consecutive cases after termination of hydatidiform mole by evacuation, curettage or hysterectomy, 13 were given prophylactic chemotherapy. One patient was not so treated because her urinary gonadotrophins (Prognosticon and mouse uterine weight tests) were under 80 I.U. per 24 hours following evacuation. Eleven patients were treated with one to three intermittent courses of methotrexate (100 mg. per course over a period of 5 days for patients with an average weight of 100 lbs. or 45 kg), with the usual care taken in the assessment of functions of the bone marrow, liver and kidney and other toxic effects. Chemotherapy was promptly discontinued as soon as the urinary gonadotrophins were less than 100 I.U. per 24 hours. No further treatment was given and these 11 patients together with the first one are well now (minimum period of 3 months to a maximum of 9 months observation). They are still being followed up at monthly intervals for assessment of urinary gonadotrophins, x-ray of chest and clinical examination.

The remaining 2 patients were additionally treated with 6-mercaptopurine (100 mg. daily for 5 days in each course) because of the presence of large quantities of urinary gonadotrophins following termination hydatidiform mole:

Case 1, Age 20, G 2/P 1: Two weeks after evacuation of hydatidiform mole and curettage, a nodule in the vagina was excised. The chest was clear but the urinary gonadotrophins were over 7 million I.U. per 24 hours. A histopathological examination of the evacuated tissue and curetting showed benign hydatidiform mole without typical features of choriocarcinoma except the presence of a few cells with hyperchromatic nuclei in the excised nodule. After 2 courses of combined methotrexate and 6-mercaptopurine she was well. She now menstruates regularly, her chest is still clear and the urinary gonadotrophins are less than 40 I.U. per 24 hours.

Case 2, Age 47, G 14/P 10: Following spontaneous evacuation, a hysterectomy was performed. Histopathological examination of the evacuated tissue showed benign hydatidiform mole and that of the excised uterus, necrotic decidua only. Her chest was clear but the urinary gonadotrophins were over 2 million I.U. per 24 hours. She was first given one course of methotrexate and then a second course of methotrexate together with 6-mercaptopurine. One day after completing the 2nd course a small nodule (approx. 1 cm. in diameter) appeared at the introitus near the urethra. This was excised and histopathological examination showed secondary choriocarcinoma. The chest which was clear previously, began to show vague opacity in the lower zones of both lung fields one week after the excision of the vaginal nodule and there was increased density a week later. The urinary gonadotrophins were less than 200 I.U. per 24 hours. She responded well to 2 further courses of methotrexate and 6-mercaptopurine and is still well 6 months after the last course. The urinary gonadotrophins are under 10 I.U. per 24 hours.

Discussion

Case 2 illustrates that metastatic trophoblastic tissue continues to develop into choriocarcinoma even during treatment after 2 courses (200 mg.) of methotrexate and one course (500 mg.) of 6-mercaptopurine. The lesion could only be considered benign to begin with as the evacuated tissue was benign hydatidiform mole and the excised uterus showed only necrotic decidua. The subsequent development of metastatic choriocarcinoma was not only found in the vulval nodule but it was also detectable in the lungs by the chest films taken at weekly intervals. After 2 more courses of chemotherapy she was in complete remission.

The question inevitably arises, as to whether it is justifiable to give prophylactic chemotherapy at all as the toxic effects are sometimes quite severe. Perhaps it was justifiable in Case 1 because of the

doubtful nature of the vaginal nodule in which the histopathological report was not available until days afterwards. But the fact remains that of the other 12 cases who received prophylactic chemotherapy, 11 might never have developed choriocarcinoma.

On going through the series of 265 cases of hydatidiform mole mentioned earlier it is interesting to note the significant relationship between the duration of positive biological tests (with frogs) and the incidence of subsequent development of choriocarcinoma (Table I). In general

Table I. *Time taken for biological tests to become negative after evacuation or hysterectomy to terminate hydatidiform mole*

Negative tests after termination	No. of Cases	Incidence of Choriocarcinoma	
		No.	Percentage
1 week	118	8	6.7
2 weeks	90	5	5.5
3 weeks	30	3	10
4 weeks	10	2	20
4 plus weeks	8	5	62.5
Undetermined	9	0	—
Total	265	23	

the longer the tests remained positive the higher was the incidence of choriocarcinoma. When they were still positive 4 weeks after termination of molar pregnancies, over half of them eventually developed choriocarcinoma. Thus it is seen that the persistent positive biological tests are an ominous sign which precedes the clinical or radiological evidence of choriocarcinoma. Such cases should be energetically treated with prophylactic chemotherapy. With the use of present sensitive gonadotrophin tests it is certain that more cases than shown in Table I would be found to be still positive 4 weeks after termination of molar pregnancies. With such a combination i.e. sensitive methods in the detection of urinary gonadotrophins and prophylactic use of chemotherapy the number of choriocarcinoma would certainly be markedly reduced if not completely wiped out following the termination of molar pregnancy.

Summary

Of the 14 consecutive cases following termination of molar pregnancies, 13 were given prophylactic chemotherapy, one of whom developed metastatic choriocarcinoma under treatment. That one was given 2 further courses of methotrexate and 6-mercaptopurine and went into complete remission. She is still well now after 6 months.

Previous studies showed that if chorionic gonadotrophins were positive at 4 weeks, over 62% developed choriocarcinoma if left untreated. With the present results, we consider it justifiable to give prophylactic chemotherapy only when chorionic gonadotrophins persist in the urine 4 weeks after termination of the molar pregnancy.

References

CHUN, D., BRAGA, C., CHOW, C., and LOK, L., Treatment of hydatidiform mole. *J. Obstet. Gynaec. Brit. Cwlth.* 71, 185—191 (1964).

The Effect of Methotrexate in Trophoblastic Diseases

Chien-Tien Hsu, * M. D., Tsu-Fang Wang, ** M. D., Shu-Eh Liang, ** M.D.,
Huo-Pang Hsu, ** M. D., Wei-Tung Tsai, * M. D. and Shu-Yuan Pen, * M. D.

*Department of Obstetrics and Gynecology, The First Army General Hospital,** and from the Department of Obstetrics and Gynecology, Provincial Taipei Hospital and Taipei Medical College,* Taipei, Taiwan, China*

Eleven patients with malignant trophoblastic neoplasia, six with choriocarcinoma and five with hydatidiform mole (three of them with invasive mole) were treated with methotrexate at a dose of 17.5—25 mg/daily for 2 to 5 days in repeat courses. One patient who was previously treated by hysterectomy for choriocarcinoma had no evidence of active growth at the onset of chemotherapy, but subsequently died. The remaining ten patients all had disseminated tumor and four of them exhibited signs of brain involvement. Eight patients responded by complete tumor regression and have remained free of disease on followup from 5 to 40 months. One patient died from disease and another from drug toxicity.

All four patients with suspected brain involvement responded, but one of them died from toxicity.

However, very interestingly, in this case, in the vaginal, pulmonary and cerebral metastatic lesions, lymphocyte and plasma cell infiltration and fibrosis were noted. These features are seen in homologous transplants, and might be expected but have not been previously described in choriocarcinoma.

One patient with hydatidiform mole and pulmonary metastases, subsequent to the response to treatment with methotrexate, became pregnant and gave birth to a term living baby which was normal in all respects except for polydactylism (accessary left little finger).

Methotrexate Treatment in Choriocarcinoma

(Preliminary Report)

KHE LOEN LIEM, M. D.

Department Obstetrics and Gynecology, School of Medicine
University of Indonesia, Djakarta

The frequency of choriocarcinoma [trophoblastic neoplasia — Ed.], is high in Indonesia. There are about 10 cases a year in the Department of Obstetrics and Gynecology, Djakarta.

Evaluation of the material from our department for the years 1952 through 1957 revealed the following mortality rates:

hydatidiform mole   4.2 % in 233 cases
choriocarcinoma villosum
[Invasive and/or metastatic mole—Ed.]
                    19.6 % in 26 cases
choriocarcinoma non-villosum
                    65.0 % in 17 cases
choriocarcinoma unclassified
                    71.0 % in   7 cases

Methotrexate either alone or in combination with surgery has been employed in 27 cases of choriocarcinoma [trophoblastic neoplasia] treated from October 1960 through December 1964. Twenty-one of these patients had shown clinical symptoms of metastasis: 12 patients with metastasis in the lungs, 4 patients with metastasis in the lungs and pelvis, 4 patients with metastasis in the vagina, and 3 patients with metastasis in the central nervous system.

Out of 12 patients examined by hysterograms 9 showed irregularities of the uterine cavity, suspicious for the presence of a malignant disease. The dose of methotrexate given orally varied from 75 mg to 400 mg:

Ten patients received 1 course (15 mg daily for 5 days), 13 received 2 courses, 2 received 3 courses, 1 patient received 4 courses, and 1 patient received 7 courses.

Side effects of methotrexate, such as stomatitis, pharyngitis, and diarrhea, were frequently encountered, but they were all of temporary nature. One patient showed leukopenia. None died of toxic effects of the drug.

Treatment consisted of methotrexate only, or methotrexate plus surgery. The result of treatment is shown in the following table.

The overall mortality rate of our material is 48 %. The follow-up time is still

Type of Trophoblastic Neoplasia	Mtx. only		Mtx. + Surgery		Overall	
	total	dead	total	dead	total	dead
Choriocarcinoma non-villosum	5	2	9	7	14	9
Choriocarcinoma villosum [Invasive or metastatic mole]	3	1	4	1	7	2
Unclassified	4	1	2	1	6	2
	12	4	15	9	27	13

too short and the number of patients too small to draw definite conclusions from this study. Our impression is that methotrexate therapy seems to influence the outcome of choriocarcinoma.

Acknowledgement

The author wishes to thank Lederle Company, U.S.A. for providing him the methotrexate.

Synopsis of discussion III

Drs. LI and HERTZ recalled the experience of the first three patients originally reported in whom intravenous administration of methotrexate was carried out in association with Dr. PAUL CONDIT. After the first three patients, intramuscular and oral administration of the drug was used in attempts to prolong the blood levels attained. Dr. HERTZ pointed out that following intramuscular administration it takes from 1 to 3 weeks for substantial reduction of gonadotropin titer to occur whereas earlier fall occurred following intravenous administration. He speculated this might be related to an artifactual effect of methotrexate on urinary excretion of chorionic gonadotropin, although better chemotherapeutic effect of the drug by intravenous administration in higher dose was not excluded. Possible interference of urinary methotrexate with bioassays must be considered, however, since after exceptionally large doses the drug might affect the bioassay system speciously giving a lower gonadotropin assay value.

Dr. HOLLAND stressed the desirability of considering tissue levels of drug rather than blood levels. In studies with Dr. WERKHEISER he had found serum concentrations to drop rapidly. Most of the day is spent without a detectable serum level of methotrexate. He discussed the efficacy of twice weekly parenteral methotrexate administration in both acute lymphocytic leukemia (SELAWRY et. al., 1965) and bronchogenic carcinoma (ROSS and SELAWRY, 1965). He indicated that although the regimen adopted by Drs. HERTZ and LI of five days of drug administration was successful in 50% of

patients it was not necessarily the optimal technique of administering methotrexate. Indeed further research on dose regimen in choriocarcinoma should be undertaken.

Consideration of additional factors that modify methotrexate susceptibility must include transport mechanisms for folate and methotrexate into tumor cells. The analogy with Murphy-Sturm lymphosarcoma is cogent and cells which ordinarily concentrate folate might be unusually susceptible to methotrexate. BERTINO and colleagues have described low levels of serum folate in patients with head and neck cancer presumptively from dietary insufficiency and in them exceptional toxicity was seen. The question of daily low dose methotrexate for choriocarcinoma was raised and deplored by HOLLAND. Enough information exists suggesting superiority of higher doses of methotrexate given infrequently to discourage initiation of studies with low drug dose. Possibly the patient would be exposed to risk of death from choriocarcinoma early in the disease before therapeutic effect could occur. High dose treatment must be individualized according to body weight or surface area, however, since drug concentrations vary in body fluids and a constant dose for all women would give high concentrations to some and low concentrations to others.

The chemotherapeutic index for choriocarcinoma was admittedly different from that for prophylaxis after mole, however, where acceptable toxicity would be considerably less. Dr. MANAHAN indicated he had treated women with mole prophylactically with small doses of methotrexate and in quite a few cases saw development of recrudescent trophoblastic neoplasia nonetheless. He has lately used more intensive treatment with success. Both Dr. HERTZ and Dr. MANAHAN reported that a high percentage of those patients referred as a chemotherapy failure were women who had been treated with low doses of methotrexate. There was general concensus that methotrexate should be given for choriocarcinoma in high doses although the schedule for these doses was not proven to be optimal when given four or five days in succession.

Dr. BURCHENAL related that Drs. BURKITT and OETTGEN both have observed failure of daily methotrexate treatment in children with the African lymphoma (BURKITT's tumor) whereas high dose short term methotrexate treatment produces a good chemotherapeutic effect in the early stages of the disease. Dr. BAGSHAWE cautioned against generalization of the high dose treatment. He has seen death in cerebral choriocarcinoma from high dose methotrexate treatment, presumptively from rapid tumor destruction, whereas giving 5 mg of the drug twice daily for nearly two weeks in combination with 6-mercaptopurine produced successful resolution with survival.

The significance of prophylactic treatment of mole was discussed and it was emphasized that 90 to 95 % of patients would not develop recrudescent disease or choriocarcinoma. Dr. MANAHAN emphasized, however, the uncertainty of prolonged followup and the difficulty of repetitive gonadotropin titers in under-developed countries. He indicated that the 5 to 10 % of women who would have further trophoblastic neoplasia without prophylactic treatment could be expected to develop clinically significant disease with high mortality risk before opportunity for therapeutic treatment. Thus, the basis for prophylaxis exists and appropriate controls would be necessary to determine whether a candidate treatment was effective.

Dr. CHUN presented clinical data on two patients with mole which subsequently developed into choriocarcinoma. They repeatedly responded to chemotherapy for prolonged periods during several years, with negative gonadotropin excretion and no evidence of metastasis, but subsequently relapsed. On one occasion, complete remission lasted for 2 years before a recrudescence. Dr. HERTZ recounted his five relapses following complete remission. In four patients relapse occurred prior to one year and in the fifth it was just over one year. Dr. HERTZ believes that as time proceeds patients become increasingly refractory to all forms of chemotherapy. He has treated 11 patients with advanced unresponsive trophoblastic neoplasia with a combination of chlorambucil, methotrexate, and actinomycin D and only 1 appears to have sustained complete remission. Dr. BREWER cited experience with actinomycin D in 11 patients following failure or resistance to methotrexate. Nine responded to actinomycin D and a 10th was cured by hysterectomy since she had non-metastatic disease.

References

Ross, C. A., and SELAWRY, O. S., Comparison of three dose schedules of methotrexate in lung cancer. *Proc. Amer. Ass. Cancer Res.* 6, 54 (1965).

SELAWRY, O. S., HANANIAN, J., WOLMAN, I. J., ABIR, E., CHEVALIER, L., GOURDEAU, R., DENTON, R., SAWITSKY, A., BURGERT, E. O., JR., MILLS, S. D., BLOM, J., JONES, B., PATTERSON, R. B., MCINTYRE, O. R., HAURANI, F. I., MOON, J. H., HOOGSTRATEN, B., KUNG, F. H., SHEEHE, P. R., FREI, E., III, and HOLLAND, J. F., New treatment schedule with improved survival in childhood leukemia. *J. Amer. med. Ass.* 194, 75—81 (1965).

Urinary Excretion of Gonadotropin and the Estrogens in Hydatidiform Mole and Choriocarcinoma

Bernhard Zondek, and Michael Finkelstein

Hormone Research Laboratory
Hebrew University-Hadassah Medical School
Jerusalem, Israel

Introduction

Choriocarcinoma is a malignant growth, whose mass production and excretion of gonadotropin can be utilized as a basis for early diagnosis and control of therapeutic procedures.

Zondek (1926) and Aschheim (1925) separately, and in 1927 jointly, reported remarkable changes that take place in the ovaries of infantile mice following a single intramuscular implantation of a small piece of either human or animal anterior pituitary tissue. These changes bring about a precocious sexual maturity and consist of the following chronological events: 1) follicle ripening and induction of vaginal estrus, 2) hyperemia of ovaries and hemorrhagic follicles, 3) luteinization and formation of corpora lutea. These reactions were called APR (anterior pituitary reaction) I, II and III, respectively. Independently, Smith (1926) arrived at similar results by performing multiple daily transplants of anterior pituitary into infantile rats.

These early observations led to a new concept in endocrinology, namely that the anterior pituitary gland secretes a hormone which stimulates the sex glands to produce their specific hormones, thus acting as a "hormonotropin". The changes in the ovary following the implantation of anterior pituitary tissue were ascribed to two factors. The first was the follicle ripening stimulating factor (Prolan A), later called FSH, and the second — the luteinizing factor (Prolan B), the LH.

In their early studies Zondek and Aschheim found that gonadotropin is exclusively produced by the anterior pituitary, with one exception — the placenta. This observation was based upon the "explosive" production and excretion of gonadotropin by the human female almost immediately following the nidation of the fertilized ovum. (Aschheim and Zondek 1927; 1928). However shortly afterwards Aschheim (1928), Zondek (1929) and Meyer (1930), noticed the increased excretion of urinary gonadotropin in cases of hydatidiform mole and of choriocarcinoma. Most interesting was the detection of a remarkably high level of gonadotropin in the liquid of hydatidiform mole and in the tissue of the mole and of choriocarcinoma. The estimation of gonadotropin in tissue obtained by curettage and in tumors (genital or extragenital) has been recommended as a diagnostic tool for tracing the presence of metastases or extragenital choriocarcinoma ("hormonal tissue diagnosis") (ZONDEK, 1929; 1942).

The pronounced increment in the excretion of the gonadotropin in urine in cases of hydatidiform mole and of choriocarcinoma has since been widely used as a diagnostic aid for the differentiation between mola hydatidiformis and choriocarcinoma on the one hand and pregnancy on the other. However, the observation of PHILLIPP (1931) that in a case of mola fibrosa no detectable gonadotropin was excreted in the urine called for more caution in suspected cases. This observation was later confirmed by several authors in rare cases of mole in which no chorionic gonadotropin was found in the urine.

In 1929 ZONDEK predicted and in 1930 demonstrated the urinary excretion of gonadotropin (Prolan B) in a case of choriocarcinoma of the testis. This was simultaneously confirmed by HEIDRICH et al., (1930) and soon after by many other authors. The presence of this gonadotropin in the urine of the human male is of considerable diagnostic importance, since it seems to be excreted exclusively in cases of malignant trophoblastic tumors.

In the present communication we shall report on our more recent experience on the urinary excretion of chorionic gonadotropin and of estrogens (with special reference to estriol) in cases of choriocarcinoma and hydatidiform mole, and on the diagnostic value of their simultaneous estimation.

Methods of estimation

Estimation of urinary excretion of chorionic gonadotropin and of estrogens in cases of mole and choriocarcinoma may be of significant diagnostic value, provided that the results are checked against values obtained during normal pregnancy and during the menstrual cycle. This is so,

because results which are obtained by using various methods for estimating the gonadotropins and the estrogens show considerable variations among tests and so cannot be directly compared.

1. Chorionic gonadotropin

Chorionic gonadotropin was estimated by the ovarian hyperemia test on infantile rats (FRANK and BERMAN, 1941; REIPRICH, 1933; SALMON et al., 1942; WALKER and WALKER, 1933; ZONDEK et al., 1945), using the modification of ZONDEK et al., (1945). This test has been used in our laboratory to our satisfaction with an accuracy of 99 % for about twenty years. In the present report the excretion of chorionic gonadotropin will be made in terms of hyperemia units. The estimations were made on first morning urine, and the results are expressed in hyperemia units per litre urine. One hyperemia unit is the least quantity of human chorionic gonadotropin producing a clear hyperemia in both ovaries of a rat. In our strain of rats one hyperemia unit (HU) roughly equals one I.U. of chorionic gonadotropin.

2. Estrone, estradiol-17β and estriol

The estrogens were estimated by the fluorometric method of FINKELSTEIN (FINKELSTEIN et al., 1947; 1960; FINKELSTEIN, 1952; LADANY and FINKELSTEIN, 1963). Aliquots of 24 hour urine collections were used for the estimation. Usually the estimations were performed on 10 ml urine samples. With this method about 1 μg/24 hrs each of estrone, estradiol-17β and estriol can be estimated with an accuracy of ± 10 %.

Urinary excretion of chorionic gonadotropin throughout gestation

The characteristic excretion of chorionic gonadotropin (HCG) during normal pregnancy may be summarized as follows.

At about the third week of gestation (one week after the expected but missed menstrual period) the urinary titer of HCG rises considerably and in most cases the hyperemia reaction turns positive in a range between 500—1,000 hyperemia units. One week later the test almost invariably becomes positive at

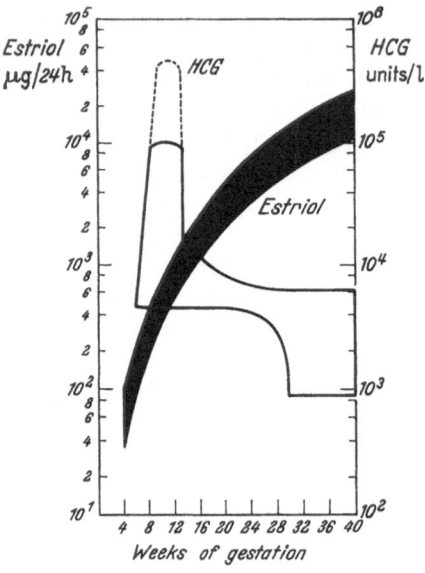

Fig. 1. Average range of excretion of HCG and estriol throughout pregnancy beginning from the 4th week of gestation

5,000 HU. In our laboratory we consider a pregnancy test positive only if the reaction is positive at 5,000 units. The excretion of gonadotropin increases significantly with the duration of pregnancy and attains its peak value between the 40th—80th day following conception. At this period, in most cases, the concentration of the HCG reaches about 100,000 HU; rarely values as high as 500,000 HU have been recorded. Following this peak period, which may last only a few days, the excretion of HCG drops in the second trimester of pregnancy to about 5,000 HU, with a further drop in the third trimester, at which time in some cases the

hyperemia reaction becomes negative at 5,000 HU and it may even turn out negative at 500 HU. Thus towards the end of pregnancy the estimation of HCG cannot be used with confidence to confirm pregnancy.

A schematic curve of excretion of HCG in pregnancy, which is composite of data obtained by several authors (Albert and Berkson, 1951; Browne and Venning, 1936; Evans et al., 1937; Laquer et al., 1943) and our own, is shown in Fig. 1.

Urinary estrogens during the menstrual cycle and in pregnancy

Three major estrogens are normally excreted in the urine of the human female during the menstrual cycle and during gestation, i. e.: estrone, estradiol-17β and estriol.

During the menstrual cycle the excretion rarely exceeds a few micrograms per 24 hour urine, the average limits being 2—20 µg for estrone, 0.5—5 µg for estradiol-17β and 2—15 µg for estriol (Finkelstein et al., 1960; Ladany and Finkelstein, 1963). These values are appreciably lower than those reported by other authors using colorimetry for the estimation (Brown, 1955).

Following conception, at about 2 weeks after the missed menstrual period the excretion of estriol rises to an average of 40—100 µg/24 hrs urine. Thus already at this period a clear distinction can be made between pregnant women and non-pregnant women who are menstruating normally (Finkelstein et al., 1960; Zondek and Finkelstein, 1962). The increase in excretion of estriol continues gradually with the progress of pregnancy attaining an average of 200—400 µg per 24 hour urine in the 8th week of gestation, 500—1,000 µg in 12th week, and so on up to an average of 10—25 mg towards the 38th week of gestation. Following delivery there is an immediate drop in the excretion of estriol, and usually after two or three days less than 100 μg in 24 hrs is excreted.

The average urinary excretion of estriol is illustrated in Fig. 1.

Since estriol is the major estrogen of pregnancy its estimation seems to be the most suitable for comparative studies in moles and in chariocarcinoma.

Urinary excretion of chorionic gonadotropin and of estriol in cases of hydatidiform mole

Results on the simultaneous estimation of chorionic gonadotropin and estriol in representative and uncomplicated cases of hydatidiform mole are compiled in Table I.

The common feature of all these cases, except one (case R. K.), is the relatively high level of chorionic gonadotropin (100,000—1,000,000 HU/l). However most of the cases were investigated close to the "peak period" of excretion of chorionic gonadotropin (i. e. 45th—80th day after conception). Therefore, in all of them with the titer of gonadotropin up to 500,000 HU the presence of a mole could not be established with certainty solely on the basis of the gonadotropin estimation.

The simultaneous estimation of estriol showed, with the exception of case D. B., that its level was much below the expected values in normal pregnancy. For instance, in the case K. S. in the twentieth week of gestation, the excretion of estriol was 166 μg/24 hrs urine. In normal pregnancy in the corresponding period of gestation the titer should be at least 1,000 μg/24 hrs urine (Fig. 1). Thus in this case both the highly elevated gonadotropin (one million HU) and the low estrogen, pointed to a molar degeneration of the placenta. However, we encountered a case (patient D. B., twelfth week gestation), where the

level of estriol was within the upper limits of the average excretion in the corresponding period of gestation (900 μg/24 hrs), and the titer of gonadotropin was elevated to 100,000 HU. Following spontaneous abortion, a histo-pathological examination revealed a partial mole.

The case R. K. deserves special consideration. Here the excretion of the chorionic gonadotropin was 5,000 HU.

Table I. *Urinary HCG and estriol in 10 cases of hydatidiform mole*

Case	Week of gestation	HCG HU/l	Estriol μg/24 hrs
R. W.	6	100,000	80
	9	500,000	85
Ch. A.	8	500,000	80
R. K.	8	5,000	
	13	5,000	37
S. L.	8	100,000	
	10	500,000	45
	13	1,000,000	31
A. L.	8	500,000	90
M. Fr.	12	1,000,000	85
D. B.*	12	100,000	900
B. Na.	14	100,000	107
K. S.	20	1,000,000	166
J. M.	20	—	11

* Partial mole.

A hydatidiform mole was detected by curettage and its presence verified by histological examination. Following the curettage the titer of gonadotropin went down to 1,000 HU, but in the course of four days increased again to 5,000 HU. A second curettage was performed, and again the titer decreased to 1,000 HU, with a subsequent increase to 5,000 HU. Following a third curettage the excretion of the gonadotropin remained negative at 500 HU. After an uneventful period of about nine months a new pregnancy was diagnosed. The hyperemia test on the 43rd day after the onset of the last menstrual period was positive at 5,000 HU. Since on the grounds of clinical examinations a mole was suspected, a further titration of chorionic gonadotropin was made on the 55th day after the last menstrual period. The titer was 500,000 HU. Six days later the excretion of chorionic gonadotropin remained unchanged. Estimation of estriol in the same urine gave 70 µg/24 hrs urine, which is considered normal for this period of gestation. Three days later the excretion of the gonadotropin decreased to 100,000 HU/l and estriol increased to 87 µg per 25 hrs urine. Four weeks later the titer of estriol was 1,200 µg/24 hrs urine. All the latter values are within the average limits of excretion of both the chorionic gonadotropin and estriol in corresponding periods of normal gestation. The subsequent course of pregnancy was uneventful and terminated with delivery of a living child and normal placenta.

This case has been given special consideration since during the first pregnancy at the time of molar transformation the excretion of the chorionic gonadotropin was typical for normal pregnancy (5,000 HU). On the other hand during the subsequent normal pregnancy the excretion of chorionic gonadotropin reached 500,000 HU/l, a level which could be characteristic of a mole, and is infrequently encountered in the "peak period" of normal pregnancy. Estimation of estriol was quite instructive in this case, since its steady increasing excretion pointed to normal placental function.

In all the patients listed in Table I the excretion of HCG ceased during 2—8 weeks following the removal of the mole, and never recurred on subsequent estimations. None of these patients experienced any further complications, and thus the results of the laboratory follow-up were in full agreement with the clinical course.

More complicated were the three cases documented in Table II. In all of them the excretion of HCG persisted for several months after the removal of the mole. In two of them a lutein cyst was found but in the third one the cause of the prolonged excretion of HCG could not be determined.

Case R. E. was treated by one us (B. Z.) about 26 years ago and a clinical diagnosis was made of luteal cysts associated with hydatidiform mole (ZONDEK, 1942). In this case the excretion of HCG (3,000 HU/l urine) persisted for over three months following the expulsion of the mole and after a curettage was performed. Following a second curettage and puncture of the right cyst with aspiration of its contents the excretion of HCG ceased within one week. It may be of interest to mention that this was the first case in which chorionic gonadotropin and estrogenic activity have been found in the fluid of a lutein cyst. The concentration of the gonadotropin was about 1,700 HU, and the concentration of the estrogen (estimated by bioassay) was equal to about 200 µg estrone per liter of fluid.

This is most remarkable since in the second case of these series (S. N.)[1], where a mole was also associated with a lutein cyst, the excretion of the urinary estrogens was not increased at all above the levels characteristic for the normal menstrual cycle. In this latter case the excretion of HCG persisted in the range between 1,000—5,000 HU/l urine for six months following removal of the mole but ceased after a lutein cyst had been extirpated.

In a third case (R.L.) the excretion of HCG reached 10,000,000 HU/l (!). Following the removal of the mole an

---

[1] This case, investigated together with Dr. N. WIZNITZER, Chief of the Maternity Hospital, Hadera, will be published in detail elsewhere.

initial drop to 5,000 HU was noted but 60 days after the operation, the excretion increased again to 50,000 HU, and continued at this level for about 30 days. Then in the course of $2 \frac{1}{2}$ months the excretion gradually decreased, with no HCG excretion at the end of this period. Neither a lutein cyst nor metastases were detected in this case, but the possibility

choriocarcinoma. Had the diagnosis in this case been made dependent on the highly increased excretion of HCG, a choriocarcinoma would have been expected.

Choriocarcinoma of the uterus

The cases of choriocarcinoma of the uterus are presented in Table III. In these cases the excretion of chorionic

Table II. *Cases of hydatidiform mole with prolonged urinary excretion of HCG*

Case	Clinical course and follow up	HCG HU/l	Estriol µg/24 hrs
R. E. (18 y)	Hydatidiform mole expelled 5 months after the last menstrual period; luteal cysts found on examination	150,000	
	Serial estimation of HCG during the next 3 months	3,000 → 7,500	
	Curettage and puncture of the right cyst with aspiration of its contents 7 days later	< 500	
S. N. (24 y)	Two months after removal of hydatidiform mole	10,000	9
	Serial estimations during the 4 months following a curettage	1,000 → 5,000	12—30
	Three weeks following removal of left lutein cyst	< 500	12
R. L. (22 y)	Pregnancy, 3 months after last menstruation. Hydatidiform mole removed;	10,000,000	
	Two weeks later	5,000	
	Eight weeks after removal of mole	50,000	
	During next three months with slow regression	50,000 → 5,000	18—45
	$5 \frac{1}{2}$ months after removal of mole	< 500	

of the presence of an undetected cyst or undiscovered remnants of the mole has to be considered. The patient remained in good health and later had two normal deliveries.

The data obtained on case R. L. demonstrates that no distinction whatsoever can be made between hydatidiform mole and choriocarcinoma on the basis of quantitative excretion of chorionic gonadotropin. This patient excreted 10 million hyperemia units of chorionic gonadotropin per liter urine. Such a high excretion is seldom seen even in a case of

gonadotropin varied from levels encountered normally in pregnancy, i. e. 5,000—10,000 (Case N. Hb.) to 1,000,000 (Cases N. H., J. R., Z. S.). Thus these results further show that by estimating urinary HCG no differential diagnosis can be made between hydatidiform mole and choriocarcinoma. The excretion of estriol was invariably low, and in the ranges characteristic for the menstrual cycle. Even so, the combined estimation of chorionic gonadotropin and of estriol cannot be used with great confidence for the differentiation between mole and

Table III. *Urinary HCG and estriol in cases of choriocarcinoma of the uterus*

Case	Clinical course and follow up	HCG HU/l	Estriol µg/24 hrs
N. Hb. (44 y)	Ten days after spontaneous abortion of hydatidiform mole	500	
	Two weeks later	1,000	
	Serial weekly estimations of HCG & estriol	5,000 → 10,000	6—21
	Hysterectomy & methotrexate (625 mg)	< 500	7—12
	Full recovery (3 years)		
N. H. (21 y)	Choriocarcinoma, 40 days after delivery complicated by expulsion of incomplete placenta	1,000,000	15
	Hysterectomy & methotrexate (625 mg)	< 500	7—12
	Full recovery (7 years)		
T. T. (23 y)	Uterine bleeding three months following abortion of hydatidiform mole	20,000	15
	Choriocarcinoma found by curettage		
	Hysterectomy & treatment with methotrexate (625 mg)	< 500	
	Full recovery (4 years)		
J. R. (34 y)	Choriocarcinoma diagnosed 6 months following delivery; Brain metastases detected	100,000	10
	Following hysterectomy and nitrogen mustard, regression of gonadotropin excretion	5,000 → 500	
	One month later & during the next 3 months Patient died	50,000 → 1,000,000	9
A. M. (42 y)	Choriocarcinoma, 3 years following hydatidiform mole		
	Hormonal assay started 6 weeks after commencement of treatment with methotrexate	5,000	15
	Serial estimations during next 4 months Patient died	5,000 → 10,000	7—18
Z. S. (50 y)	Choriocarcinoma, one year after curettage for hydatidiform mole & three months following removal of lutein cysts; Metastases found in the lungs	1,000,000	9
	Hysterectomy & methotrexate		
	Serial estimations during 20 months Patient died	5,000 → 500,000	7—15

choriocarcinoma of the uterus, because in some of our cases of hydatidiform mole the excretion of estriol was low as in the cases of choriocarcinoma.

Estimation of chorionic gonadatropin is an excellent aid for following the efficacy of treatment in cases of choriocarcinoma (Table III). It can be seen that in cases N. Hb., N. H., T. T., following hysterectomy and chemotherapy the excretion of HCG dropped to undetectable levels, and the clinical course proved highly satisfactory. On the other hand in cases J. R., Z. S. and A. M. the excretion of HCG did never diminish entirely, and all of them proved fatal.

Choriocarcinoma of the testis and of the ovary

These cases are shown in Table IV. The single case of choriocarcinoma of the testis excreted 1,000 HU chorionic gonadotropin per liter urine. The characteristic feature in this case was the high excretion of estriol (470 µg/24 hrs). Although this figure was obtained by the older method for estimation of estriol, and is probably an overestimate, the corrected value, based on our experience with both new and old methods, would be no less than 400 µg/24 hrs. The usual range of excretion of estriol in normal human male is about 1—5 µg/24 hrs urine. The elevated excretion of urinary estrogens in cases of choriocarcinoma of the testis was noted by HAMBURGER (1958) in about 40% of an extensive series of patients. The results in our case are in accord with his observations.

In contrast, in the two cases of choriocarcinoma of the ovary the excretion of estriol was not increased. In one of them (Case R. F.) the excretion of HCG was in the range characteristic for choriocarcinoma of the uterus (2,000,000 HU), but in the other (Case C. K.) it was increased only to 500 HU. Nevertheless this increased excretion of HCG proved of high diagnostic value and led to the correct diagnosis of malignancy.

The high excretion of estrogens in the case of choriocarcinoma of the testis, and their non-increase in cases of choriocarcinoma of the ovary seems incompatible at first sight. This apparently paradoxical result can be explained, however, by the following reasoning:

It is known that HCG may stimulate the testis in vivo to produce steroid hormones, and inter alia the estrogens (PINCUS, 1958). In choriocarcinoma of the testis the tumor produces chorionic gonadotropin, and the latter may stimulate the production of estrogens by the testicular

tissue. Conversely, HCG per se (without previous stimulation with FSH) has little or no stimulating properties on the production of the estrogens by the ovary in vivo (GEMZELL et al., 1958). Thus the chorionic gonatropin produced by choriocarcinoma of the uterus or of the ovary does not induce an increase in the estrogens secretion by the ovary.

Alternatively, the low urinary estrogens in our cases of ovarian choriocarcinoma could be due to the unrespon-

Table IV. *Urinary HCG and estrone, estradiol-17β and estriol in choriocarcinoma of testis and of ovary*

Case	Clinical course	HCG HU/l	Estriol µg/24 hrs
F. (24 y. m.)	Patient died	1,000	470
R. F. 11 6/12 y. f.)	Patient died	1,000,000	5.5
C. K. (9 y. f.)	Patient died	500	4.0

siveness of the infantile ovary (the patients being 9 and 11 years old, respectively) to stimulation by HCG.

Conclusions

In most cases of mole, HCG is excreted in the urine in quantities exceeding those excreted in pregnancy. The estimations should be performed on a serial basis, and the results should be carefully compared with those obtained in normal pregnancies. Care should be especially exerted during the "peak period" of excretion of HCG between the 40th—80th day of gestation. Since this "peak period" is rather short, and lasts no longer than one to two weeks, several estimations of gonadotropin are recommended as a guide for the correct diagnosis. The high excretion of HCG usually persists a few weeks following the removal of the mole.

This is in contrast to normal pregnancy, where normally one week after delivery, no chorionic gonadotropin is excreted any longer in the urine. In isolated cases the excretion of chorionic gonadotropin may continue for several months after the expulsion of the mole. In such cases a careful search for lutein cysts and/or choriocarcinoma should be made.

Parallel estimations of estriol may be most helpful and auxiliary to the estimation of gonadotropin. Since in normal pregnancy the excretion of estriol increases with the progress of gestation, but usually does not increase considerably in cases of mole, serial estimations showing an increase in the excretion of chorionic gonadotropin, but an arrest or even a decrease in the excretion of estriol, point to degenerative changes in the placenta. In most cases of hydatidiform mole the excretion of estriol is higher than during the menstrual cycle, but lower than in the corresponding week of gestation. Occasionally cases of hydatidiform mole may be encountered excreting estriol in quantities comparable to normal pregnancy. This may be especially so in cases of partial mole.

Choriocarcinoma of the uterus cannot be distinguished from mole merely by estimating chorionic gonadotropin. In both cases the quantities of excreted chorionic gonadotropin may be in similar ranges. In most cases of choriocarcinoma the excretion of estriol is not increased above the levels normally found during the menstrual cycle, and it is usually lower than in hydatidiform mole. The low excretion of estriol in choriocarcinoma cannot serve for a differential diagnosis from a mole, however, because some of the cases of mole may also show a comparably low excretion of estriol.

Choriocarcinoma of the testis may be characterized by the high excretion of both HCG and estrogens. On the other hand in choriocarcinoma of the ovary excretion of HCG is not accompanied by an increase in the urinary estrogens. The difference in the estrogen excretion between choriocarcinoma of the testis and that of the uterus or of the ovary may be explained by the stimulating property of HCG on steroid biosynthesis in the testis which is not pronounced in the case of the ovary.

Acknowledgement

The skilled assistance of Mrs. L. BEYTH and Mrs. V. PFEIFFER is gratefully acknowledged.

References

ALBERT, A., and BERKSON, J., A clinical bioassay for chorionic gonadotropin. *J. clin. Endocr.* 11, 805—820 (1951).

ASCHHEIM, S., Über die Funktion des Ovariums. *Z. Geburtsh. Gynäk.* 90, 387—392 (1926).

— Über Luteincystenbildung im Ovarium bei Blasenmole und Chlorionepithelioma malignum. Die Entstehung dieser Luteincysten durch Wirkung des Hypophysenvorderlappeninkrets. *Zbl. Gynäk.* 52, 602—609 (1928).

ASCHEIM, S., u. ZONDEK, B., Hypophysenvorderlappenhormon und Ovarialhormon im Harn von Schwangeren. *Klin. Wschr.* 6, 1322 (1927).

—, — Schwangerschaftsdiagnose aus dem Harn durch Hormonnachweis). *Klin. Wschr.* 7, 8—9 (1928).

BROWN, J. B., A chemical method for the determination of oestriol, oestrone and oestradiol in human urine. *Biochem. J.* 60, 185—193 (1955).

BROWNE, J. S. L., and VENNING, E. H., Excretion of gonadotropic substances in the urine during pregnancy. *Lancet 1936 II.* 1507—1511.

EVANS, H. M., KOHLS, C. L., and WONDER, D. H., Gonadotropic hormone in the blood and urine of early pregnancy; the normal occurence of transient extremely high levels. *J. Amer. med. Ass.* 108, 287—289 (1937).

FINKELSTEIN, M., Fluorometric determination of micro amounts of oestrone-oestradiol and oestriol in urine. *Acta endocr. (Kbh.)* 10, 149—166 (1952).

— HESTRIN, S., and KOCH, W., Estimation of steroid estrogen by fluorimetry. *Proc. Soc. exp. Biol. (N. Y.)* 64, 64—71 (1947).

— JEWELEWICZ, R., KLEIN, O., PFEIFER, V., and SODMORIA-BECK, S., *Prenatal Care,* p. 12—27 Groningen, The Netherlands: P. Noordhoff, Ltd. 1960.

FRANK, R. T., and BERMAN, R. L., A twenty-four hour pregnancy test. *Amer. J. Obstet. Gynec.* 42, 492—496 (1941).

GEMZELL, C. A., DICZFALUSY, E., and TILLINGER, G., Clinical effect of human pituitary follicle-stimulating hormone (FSH). *J. clin. Endocr.* 18, 1333—1348 (1958).

HAMBURGER, C., Gonadotrophins, androgens and oestrogens in cases of malignant tumours of the testes. Ciba Found. Coll. on Endocrinol. 12, 200—207 (1958).

HEIDRICH, L., FELS, E. u. MATHIAS, E., Testikulares Chorionepitheliom mit Gynäkomastie und mit einigen Schwangerschaftserscheinungen gleichzeitig ein Beitrag zur Pathologie der hormonal-aktiven Gewächse. *Bruns' Beitr. klin. Chir.* 150, 349 bis 384 (1930).

LADANY, S., and FINKELSTEIN, M., Isolation of estrone, 17 B-estradiol and estriol from female human urine. *Steroids* 2, 297—318, (1963).

LAQUER, F., DOETL, K., u. FRIEDRICH, H., *Medizin u. Chemie* 2, 117 (1943).

MEYER, R., *Zbl. Gynäk.* 54, 587—593 (1930).

PHILIPP, E., Die Wirkung von Hypothysenvorderlappen und von Placenta auf die Uterusschleimhaut beim Kaninchen. *Zbl. Gynäk.* 55, 929—941 (1931).

PINCUS, G., Ciba Found. Coll. on Endocrinol. 12, 212—214 (1958).

REIPRICHT, W., Eine neue Schwangerschafts-Schnell-Reaktion aus dem Harn („30-Stunden-Reaktion"). *Klin. Wschr.* 12, 1441 bis 1444 (1933).

SALMON, U. J., GEIST, S. H., FRANK, I. L., POOLE, C., and SALMON, A. A., A rapid pregnancy test (2—6 hours). Endocrinology 30, 1039 (1942).

SMITH, P. E., Hastening development of female genital system by daily homoplastic-pituitary transplants. *Proc. Soc. exp. Biol. (N. Y.)* 24, 131—132 (1926).

WALKER, T. F., and WALKER, D. V. H., A modification of the Aschheim-Zondek test. *J. Amer. med. Ass.* 111, 1460 (1933).

ZONDEK, B., Über die Funktion des Ovariums. *Z. Geburtsh. Gynäk.* 90, 372—380 (1926).

— Hypophysenvorderlappen und Schwangerschaft. *Endokrinologie* 5, 425—434 (1929).

— Qualitative und quantitative Gewebsuntersuchung auf Hypophysenvorderlappenhormon nach Gewebsentgiftung. Bedeutung für die Diagnose des Chorionepitheliomas. *Zbl. Gynäk.* 54, 2306—2308 (1930).

— Versuch einer biologischen (hormonalen) Diagnostik beim malignen Hodentumor. *Chirurg* 2, 1072 (1930).

— Importance of increased production and excretion of gonadotropic hormone for diagnosis of hydatidiform mole. *J. Obstet. Gynaec. Brit. Emp.* 49, 397—411 (1942).

—, u. ASCHHEIM, S., Hypophysenvorderlappen und Ovarium. Beziehungen der endokrinen Drüsen zur Ovarialfunktion. *Arch. Gynäk.* 130. 1—45 (1927).

—, e FINKELSTEIN, M., Studies on urinary estrogens with special reference to estriol. *Scritti in onore del prof. Giuseppe Tesauro,* p. 2333—2346, ed. Montanino. Napoli 1962.

—, SULMAN, F., and BLACK, R., The hyperemia effect of gonadotropins on the ovary and its use in a rapid pregnancy test. *J. Amer. med. Ass.* 128, 939—944 (1945).

Endocrinological Studies Relating to Trophoblastic Disease in Man

Roy Hertz, M. D., Ph. D.

Endocrinology Branch, National Cancer Institute, Bethesda, Maryland

Mammalian trophoblast is among the very earliest tissues to differentiate during ontogenetic development. It is therefore of singular significance that trophoblastic cells in several primate species are known to produce hormones. We shall be concerned here only with those hormonally active substances known to be produced by tumors containing trophoblastic elements. Such hormone-producing trophoblastic tumors have been identified with regularity and certainty only in man. Scattered cases of choriocarcinoma in the dog are reported in the veterinary literature, but the hormonal activity of such rare canine tumors has not been clearly established. The teratoid testicular tumors of mice described by Stevens and Little (1954) apparently are not hormone-producing.

For all practical purposes, then, man is the only known natural host for the type of tumor to be discussed here.

We shall be mainly concerned with the spectrum of variably malignant tumors which arises in the human fetal chorion. This includes hydatidiform mole, chorioadenoma destruens [invasive mole-Ed.], and choriocarcinoma. These respective lesions are observed to evolve clinically from a fetal chorion in an unpredictable temporal progression (Hertz, et al., 1964. Accordingly, we refer to these chorionic tumors collectively as "trophoblastic disease" [trophoblastic neoplasia-Ed.].

In addition, hormone-producing teratoid tumors containing trophoblastic elements arise in numerous sites in adults and children of both sexes. The ovaries and the testes are frequent sites for the origin of these tumors, but they are noted also to arise presumably from embryonal rests in the mediastinum, in the preaortic region or in such viscera as the liver. The common property of such tumors is that they contain trophoblastic elements which, however, are not always readily identifiable in routine morphological analysis.

Our clinical and chemotherapeutic studies on these tumors have been described elsewhere and will be alluded to here only in their endocrinological aspects (Hertz et al., 1964; Hertz et al., 1961).

The primary hormonal product of the trophoblastic tumors of man is chorionic gonadotropin. Zondek first demonstrated biological effects of this substance not only in normal pregnancy but also in the urine and blood of both men and women with trophoblastic tumors. The presence of this hormone is demonstrable by several biological assays which have varying degress of sensitivity. Nevertheless, our clinical experience has demonstrated that the most sensitive and perhaps least specific of these tests, namely the mouse uterine weight test, when applied to an appropriately prepared concentrate from a 24-hour urine specimen of a patient with trophoblastic disease serves as a valid index of the presence of residual trophoblastic tumor tissue.

Table I lists the relative sensitivity of the various biological tests for the presence of gonadotropin in human urine or serum. It will be noted that the mouse uterine weight response requires less chorionic type of gonadotropin than any other response. Hence we have found it to be most useful in detecting small amounts of residual hormone-producing tissue in man. Great care must be exercised in the quantitative reaction and concentration of the active material from body fluids. Also the test mice must be genetically standardized and maintained under the most rigorous standards of sanitation and nutrition.

With these precautions we have experienced reasonably good control in monitoring our chemotherapeutic efforts. We have relied on this test during eight years' experience in treating 121 patients with metastatic trophoblastic disease and 40 patients with non-metastatic trophoblastic disease. Among 120 cases in which our laboratory data had previously indicated complete absence of residual disease subsequent clinical or hormonal evidence of relapse occurred in only seven instances.

It should be emphasized that quantitative control of chemotherapy of trophoblastic disease is no better than the quality and sensitivity of the chorionic gonadotropin assays applied to properly collected and prepared specimens.

The endocrinological effects of the gonadotropin produced by the tumor on the patient are of interest. Thus trophoblast-containing tumors arising in children are associated in some instances with sexual precocity (JOLLY, 1955). This indicates that the gonadotropin can effectively activate the immature gonad of the host. In women with hydatidiform mole or choriocarcinoma, one observes clinical evidence of marked bilateral ovarian enlargement in approximately 30 % of the cases during the initial phase of the disease process. The ovarian enlargement is frequently extreme, representing a 10- to 20-fold increase over normal ovarian size. These huge ovaries are made up of very large follicular cysts, some of which have become highly hemorrhagic. Ovulation is not noted, but substantial thecal luteinization occurs in a large proportion of the follicular cysts. Following the removal of the hydatidiform mole, these

Table I. *Minimal effective dose of chorionic gonadotropin for varios target organ responses*

Response	M. E. D.
Mouse uterine weight	0.1 I.U.
Rat ovarian hyperemia	0.5 I.U.
Rat uterine weight	0.5 I.U.
Rat ventral prostate weight	0.25 I.U.
Rabbit ovulation	3—5 I.U.
Toad or frog sperm	25 I. U.

enlarged ovaries revert to normal size in the course of two to three months and normal cyclic function and fertility are observed. However, in those cases which progress to chorioadenoma destruens or choriocarcinoma, the same ovarian involution is observed despite the continued presence of enormous titers of chorionic gonadotropin in the host as evidenced by bioassay on blood and urine. Thus, in thirty of our patients who have come to autopsy with extensive metastatic trophoblastic disease and with associated high gonadotropin titers, in no instance did the ovaries reflect any gonadotropic effect of the hormone present. Hence, we are led to the inference that there develops some degree of refractoriness to chorionic gonadotropin stimulation on the part of the previously responsive ovary. The plasma of patients who have survived this process of initial ovarian stimulation and whose total gonadotropin titers have returned to normal levels do not possess the capacity to inhibit chorionic gonadotropin as tested by the mouse uterine or rat ovarian weight methods. Hence this remarkable loss of sensivity to an isologous protein hormone remains a phenomenon for further investigation.

Conversely, twelve of our patients who have been incompletely cleared of metastatic trophoblastic disease and who have continued to exhibit substantial residual titers of chorionic hormone have exhibited normal cyclic menstruation for periods up to one year while in incomplete remission from their disease. It would seem then that the human ovary can respond to endogenous pituitary gonadotropin while exhibiting complete refractoriness to chorionic gonadotropin of tumor origin. We have found, however, that the anterior pituitary of seven women dying with huge titers of chorionic hormone in their blood and urine contained normal amounts of gonadotropin as evidenced by bioassay. The mechanism whereby these gonadal effects are produced merits further study.

A related phenomenon is observed in such patients with metastatic trophoblastic disease in incomplete remission. Such patients exhibit a remarkable quantitative constancy in the residual gonadotropin titers encountered. Urinary titers before therapy may vary between 20,000,000 and 100,000 mouse uterine units per 24 hours. However, initial response to chemotherapy when associated with the development of drug resistance is accompanied by a narrow range of urinary titers of from 2,000 to 5,000 mouse uterine units per 24 hours in 75% of the cases. These patients maintain this narrow range of titers for periods varying 3 months to 2 years, frequently with no other manifestation of residual disease. However, recrudescence of the disease process may be anticipated in all such cases unless they are successfully treated with a second ef-

fective drug. From an endocrinological point of view, the constancy of the residual titers in such cases is remarkable and its biological significance remains obscure.

In adult male patients with testicular tumors which are productive of very large amounts of chorionic gonadotropin, there is no evidence of gonadotropic stimulation of the contralateral testis. Thus the ketosteroid excretion levels in 25 such patients have been found to be within normal limits. Leydig-cell hyperplasia is observed only in a few cases in that portion of the involved testis which is immediately adjacent to the hormone-producing tumor mass. Nevertheless, some degree of derangement in steroid function is suggested by the occurrence of gynecomastia in some of these cases. The apparent refractoriness of the testis of the host to tumor chorionic gonadotropin is in direct contrast to the known responsiveness of the testis of the normal adult male to chorionic gonadotropin prepared from the urine of normally pregnant women.

Such discrepancies have led us to an exhaustive comparison of the biological and immunological properties of chorionic gonadotropin derived from the urine of pregnant women and that prepared from the urine of women with metastatic trophoblastic disease. We have been unable to detect any significant differences by the following criteria: (a) dose-response curves in both the mouse uterine weight test and the rat ovarian weight tests; (b) augmentation effects on rat ovarian weight response to ovine F. S. H. (follicle stimulating hormone); (c) inhibition of rat ovarian weight response to tumor or pregnancy chorionic gonadotropin by antisera prepared with either type of hormone as antigen; (d) immunoassay of biologically equivalent amounts of tumor or pregnancy hormone when tested for agglutination inhibition employing antisera prepared against either antigen; (e) identity of behavior in immunodiffusion tests in Ouchterlony plates (LEWIS, *et. al.,* 1964). By all of these criteria no distinct differentiation between hormone from these two sources could be made.

However, REISFELD, *et. al.,* (1959) have described a difference in the behavior in electrophoresis of the hormonal activity of the plasma of pregnant women and that of women with metastatic trophoblastic disease. In these studies the biological activity of the serum of twelve pregnant women was found to be largely in the gamma globulin fraction with relatively little in the beta globulin fraction. However, in the serum of patients with metastatic trophoblastic disease, the activity was found almost entirely in the beta globulin fraction with very little in the alpha globulin fraction. These findings reflect a difference in the transport of the hormonal activity in these two states but may not necessarily indicate a chemical difference between the hormones produced.

The association of hydatidiform mole with clinical evidence of thyrotoxicosis has been recognized for some time. Since both these diseases occur somewhat selectively in young women, it has been difficult to determine whether or not this phenomenon is to be attributed to coincidence. In our experience with 93 patients with metastatic trophoblastic disease in whom the customary parameters of thyroid function were studied, we encountered seven women with laboratory evidence of increased thyroid function (ODELL, *et. al.,* 1963). Assay of tumor tissue from two of these patients by Dr. BATES revealed the presence of T. S. H. in amounts greatly exceeding that found in blood. In two other patients elevated plasma levels of T. S. H. were demonstrable. Moreover, in 3 of these patients the suppression of the disease by the folic acid antagonist Methotrexate was accompanied by a prompt return of their thyroid function tests to normal without specific antithyroid therapy. Hence, it would appear that certain trophoblastic tumors produce thyrotropin as well as gonadotropin.

It should be emphasized in closing that trophoblastic disease is only one example of the numerous hormone-producing tumors of man which provide such specific indicators of tumor activity. It may be anticipated that such unique indicators will prove of great significance not only in chemotherapeutic studies but in our further comprehension of the nature of neoplastic disease generally.

Reference

HERTZ, R., LEWIS, J., and LIPSETT, M. B., Five years' experience with the chemotherapy of metastatic choriocarcinoma and related trophoblastic tumors in women. *Amer. J. Obstet. Gynec.* **82**, 631—640 (1961).

— Ross, G. T., and LIPSETT, M. B., Chemotherapy in women with trophoblastic disease: choriocarcinoma, chorioadenoma destruens, and complicated hydatidiform mole. *Ann. N. Y. Acad. Sci.* **114**, 881—885 (1964).

JOLLY, H., Sexual precocity. Springfield, Ill.: Thomas, 1955.

LEWIS, J., DRAY, S., GENUTH, S., and SCHWARTZ, H. S., Demonstration of immunological similarities of human pregnancy gonadotropin and choriocarcinoma gonadotropin with antisera prepared in rabbits and monkeys *J. clin. Endocr.* **24**, 197—204 (1964).

ODELL, W. D., BATES, R. W., RIVLIN, R. S., LIPSETT, M. B., and HERTZ, R., Increased thyroid function without clinical hyperthyroidism in patients with choriocarcinoma. *J. clin. Endocrin.* **23**, 658—664 (1963).

REISFELD, R. A., BERGENSTAL, D. M., and HERTZ, R., Distribution of gonadotropic hormone activity in the serum proteins of normal pregnant women and patients with trophoblastic tumors. *Arch. Biochem.* **81**, 456—463 (1959).

STEVENS, L. C., and LITTLE, C. C., Spontaneous testicular teratomas in an inbred strain of mice. *Proc. nat. Acad. Sci.* (Wash.) **40**, 1080—1087 (1954).

Pelvic Angiography in the Management of Malignant Trophoblastic Disease

J. P. de V. Hendrickse, M. B., Ch. B., D. C. H., M. R. C. O. G.,
W. Peter Cockshott, M. D., D. M. R. D., Ed.,
and Dinah M. James, M. Pharm, Ph. D.

*Departments of Obstetrics & Gynaecology, Radiology and Pharmacology,
University of Ibadan, Ibadan, Nigeria*

Pelvic angiography in the management of malignant trophoblastic disease

One-hundred pelvic angiograms were performed between 1961 and 1964 at University College Hospital Ibadan during the investigation of malignant trophoblastic disease [neoplasia – Ed.] (M. T. D.). Fifty-seven examinations were performed to establish the diagnosis, which was confirmed in 41 patients. Twenty-six of these patients had a total of 43 followup angiograms while under treatment.

Previous communications from this hospital have described the use of pelvic angiography in the diagnosis of trophoblastic tumours (Cockshott, *et al.,* 1964; Hendrickse, *et. al.,* 1964). This communication describes certain further clinical and diagnostic features, and discusses the value of serial pelvic angiography in patients receiving chemotherapy.

Advantages of pelvic angiography

Uterine curettage in patients with suspected M. T. D. carries the risk of disseminating the growth and causing tumour-tissue emboli to reach the lungs. Furthermore, curettage may produce such severe haemorrhage that emergency hysterectomy may be necessary — a procedure which is nowadays otherwise seldom indicated in cases of M. T. D. as a result of the success of chemotherapy. Apart from the direct hazards of diagnostic curettage in this condition, the interpretation of the findings may be difficult, a negative histological report may merely mean that the tumour does not communicate with the uterine cavity and has therefore been missed by the curette.

We have found pelvic angiography to be a very useful diagnostic procedure when the disease has been suspected clinically, and raised chorionic gonadotropin levels have been found in the urine. Indeed, M. T. D. has been demonstrated by pelvic angiography in 5 patients with histologically normal curettings.

Angiographic appearance of M. T. D.

A constant feature of the arteriogram of patients with pelvic desposits of M. T. D. is dilatation of the vessels supplying the uterus and the adnexa. The initial films show enlargement of one or both uterine arteries to beyond 1 millimetre in diameter: the ovarian arteries may also be enlarged. The uterine arteries may show an increase in the amount of redundant coilings, particularly before they reach the lateral border of the uterus. (Fig. 1 a, b.) The degree of separation of the uterine arteries and the length of the ascending portion along the lateral borders of the uterus indicates the size of the pillary staining is barely discernable. (Fig. 1 c, d.)

In most cases of M. T. D. a functional arterio-venous shunt develops through the tumour deposits, and sometimes this may be sufficiently developed for contrast to appear in efferent veins in the early phase of the examination when the arteries are

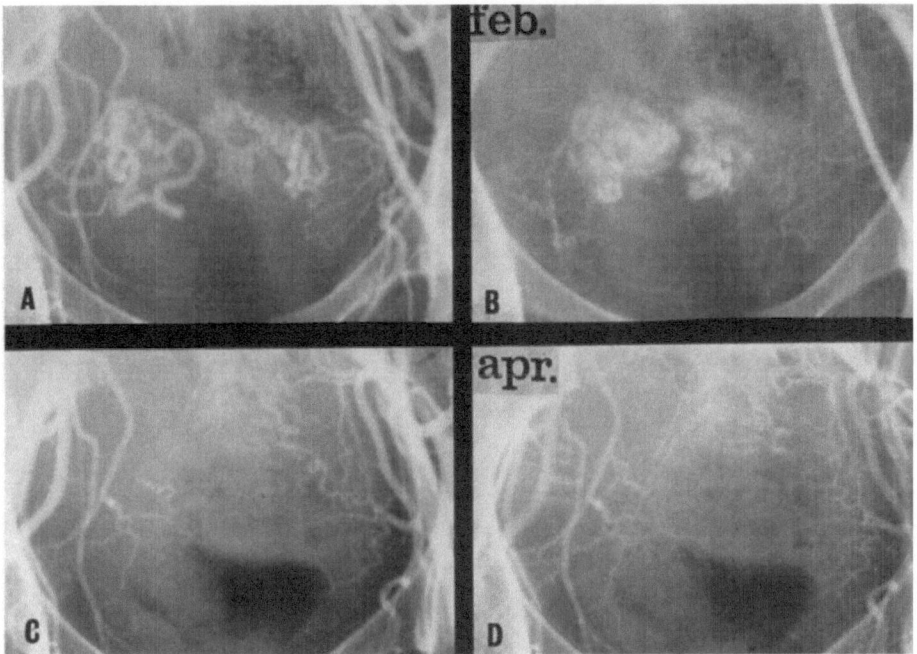

Fig. 1. Initial arteriogram. A Arterial phase showing enlarged redundant uterine arteries and prominent spiral myometrial branches. B Later phase showing spiral vessels emptying into irregular vascular spaces. *Nine weeks later* after therapy. C and D Return to normal. The uterine arteries are small and the vascular spaces are no longer apparent

uterus. In M.T.D. the spiral myometrial vessels are much more obvious than normal and they may be considerably enlarged.

Their ramifications provide further radiological evidence of the position and size of the uterus. (Fig. 1, 2, 3.) In later films, contrast medium is seen to enter ill-defined irregular vascular spaces which remain opacified throughout the period of study. In this phase of an angiogram of a normal non-pregnant uterus, ca-

still opacified. Such gross arterio-venous shunts have been seen in 5 patients.

Parametrial extension, pelvic and vaginal secondary deposits may be demonstrated by angiography. On some occasions vaginal secondaries failed to fill with contrast — perhaps because of their necrotic state. On the other hand we have twice demonstrated foci of tumour in the region of the vagina and bladder that could not be detected by clinical examination. The early films in such cases show

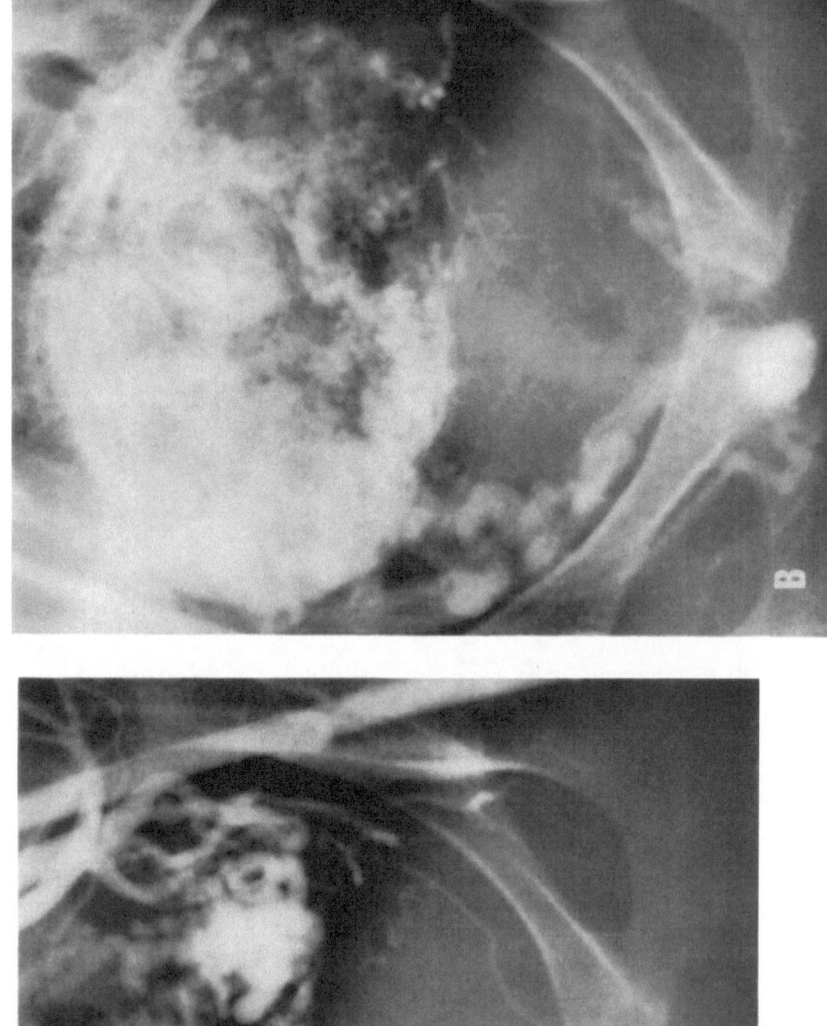

Fig. 2. A An early arterial phase. Bilateral large uterine vessels draining at once into vascular spaces that communicate with veins. A secondary deposit overlying the pubis is seen to be filling.

B A later phase reveals a large uterus, many dilated spiral branches and A. V. shunting through the secondary deposit dilatation of the obturator, pudendal or other pelvic vessels. (Fig. 2.)

Difficulties of Interpretation

There are other conditions that may show angiographic features resembling those of M. T. D. The history, clinical findings and especially the level of human chorionic gonadotropin (H. C. G.) excretion, must therefore be considered together with the angiographic findings before coming to a final diagnosis.

Confusion is likely to arise with missed abortion in patients who are bleeding vaginally and in whom some placental circulation persists. In such cases H. C. G. excretion levels will exclude M. T. D.

In cases of missed abortion where the placental circulation has ceased, the arteriographic features may simulate hydatidiform mole. However, the later stages of the examination do not show the characteristic widely-scattered intervillous vascular spaces.

In early pregnancy, the angiographic appearances may be confused with M. T. D., which is unfortunate because the H. C. G. levels are raised in both conditions. However, the history and physical signs, combined if necessary with serial observations in doubtful cases, should resolve the difficulty.

H. C. G. Excretion

A biological method of assay on urine using Xenopus laevis was employed here initially and this served as a fairly good guide to diagnosis and therapy. By this method, however, it was not possible to determine levels below 2000 i.u./litre. Immunological methods of assay were then studied, and a haemagglutination technique applied to concentrated extracts of urine was developed. By this method, values between 200 and 2000 i.u./litre could be measured quantitatively.

Excretion values of less than 200 i.u./litre were regarded as normal, and this was confirmed by studies on the urine from non-pregnant normal women. A report of this study will be published elsewhere.

We have already mentioned the importance of correlating angiographic findings with H. C. G. levels. BAGSHAWE (1963) emphasised that "pregnancy tests" are not sufficiently sensitive to establish a diagnosis of M. T. D. Our experience has confirmed this, since we have seen active disease in the presence of repeatedly negative pregnancy tests. Concentration methods and assay in such cases have shown the presence of low levels of H. C. G.

In every case of M. T. D., excretion values of H. C. G. were in keeping with the clinical diagnosis, even where the pelvic findings were negative.

Angiographic findings in two cases suggested M. T. D., but the H. C. G. levels were normal and a diagnosis of missed abortion was made. This was later confirmed by histological examination of uterine curettings.

Follow-up Angiography in cases under treatment

We have carried out pelvic angiographic procedures to assess the results of chemotherapy in 26 patients and three forms of response have been observed.

In thirteen the uterine, ovarian and myometrial vessels returned to a normal calibre, the uterus became smaller and the spaces were no longer evident in the arteriogram (Fig. 1).

The return of the angiographic appearances to normal coincided with clinical improvement and a fall in the level of chorionic gonadotropin excretion. In 4 patients who did not have an initial angiogram, normal appearances were found after treatment.

The five patients who had prominent arterio-venous communications at the time of their initial diagnostic examination showed a different behaviour following chemotherapy.

Freedom from active disease was indicated by absence of clinical signs and a return to normal H. C. G. excretion levels. However, the evidence of arteriovenous shunting persisted in the follow-up angiograms. Consequently the uterine arteries or more usually a single artery, remained dilated and obvious.

The myometrial vessels remained more prominent than usual, but their spiral pattern became more distinct than it was at the time of the initial diagnostic examination. The spiral vessels supplying the part of the uterus close to the site of the fistula were seen to drain directly into dilated vascular spaces.

In the initial arteriograms, contrast medium was seen to pass into a single dilated ovarian vein, but after chemotherapy a plexus of veins appeared to develop. This was probably due to filling of venous pathways by the passage of contrast from the high-pressure arterial system into the low-pressure valveless pelvic veins. This feature has been seen by us in traumatic arterio-venous fistulae, and was also described by Hol and Ingebrigsten (1960). A bruit could only be detected in one of these five patients and it remains to be seen whether the fistulae will short circuit a sufficient part of the cardiac output to cause systemic circulatory disturbances. So far the clinical findings do not indicate that this is occurring. Persistence of A. V. communications after chemotherapy and X-ray therapy has been recorded and illustrated in a case of chorionepithelioma by Highman and Sutton (1964).

The vascularity of the uterus and the free anastomosis between uterine vessels may cause difficulty in differentiation between persistent vascular spaces in a tumour and spaces filled passively through communications established after necrosis of the tumour. Once again, interpretation should be guided by the clinical progress of the patient and serial determinations of H. C. G. excretion levels.

Shunting may occur through a secondary deposit and this may equally persist following chemotherapy (Fig. 3).

The final category to be considered is that of patients who did not respond completely to chemotherapy. Three patients developed drug resistance and one patient (who interrupted her treatment) returned with a recurrence after an initial favourable response.

Where drug-resistance was present, the uterus initially showed some diminution in size but did not return to normal. The uterine arteries remained large and the spiral arteries prominent. The vascular spaces were no longer as large and obvious as formerly but during the later phases of the examination many small abnormal vessels could still be distinguished and these drained into enlarged central veins.

In the patient with recurrence the angiographic studies showed a return to the typical picture of M. T. D. after a previously normal angiogram.

The angiographic findings in this small group of patients confirmed the diagnosis of resistance and recurrence made on clinical grounds and from H. C. G. excretion studies.

Normal Pelvic Angiograms in Cases of M.T.D.

It is well known that extra-pelvic metastases of M. T. D. may occur without any evidence of a uterine primary source. (Maier and Taylor 1947, Park and Lees 1950, Acosta-Sison 1957, Richir et al 1961, Chan 1962.)

Six of our patients with proven M. T. D. were found to have normal pelvic angiograms. All had raised H. C. G. ex-

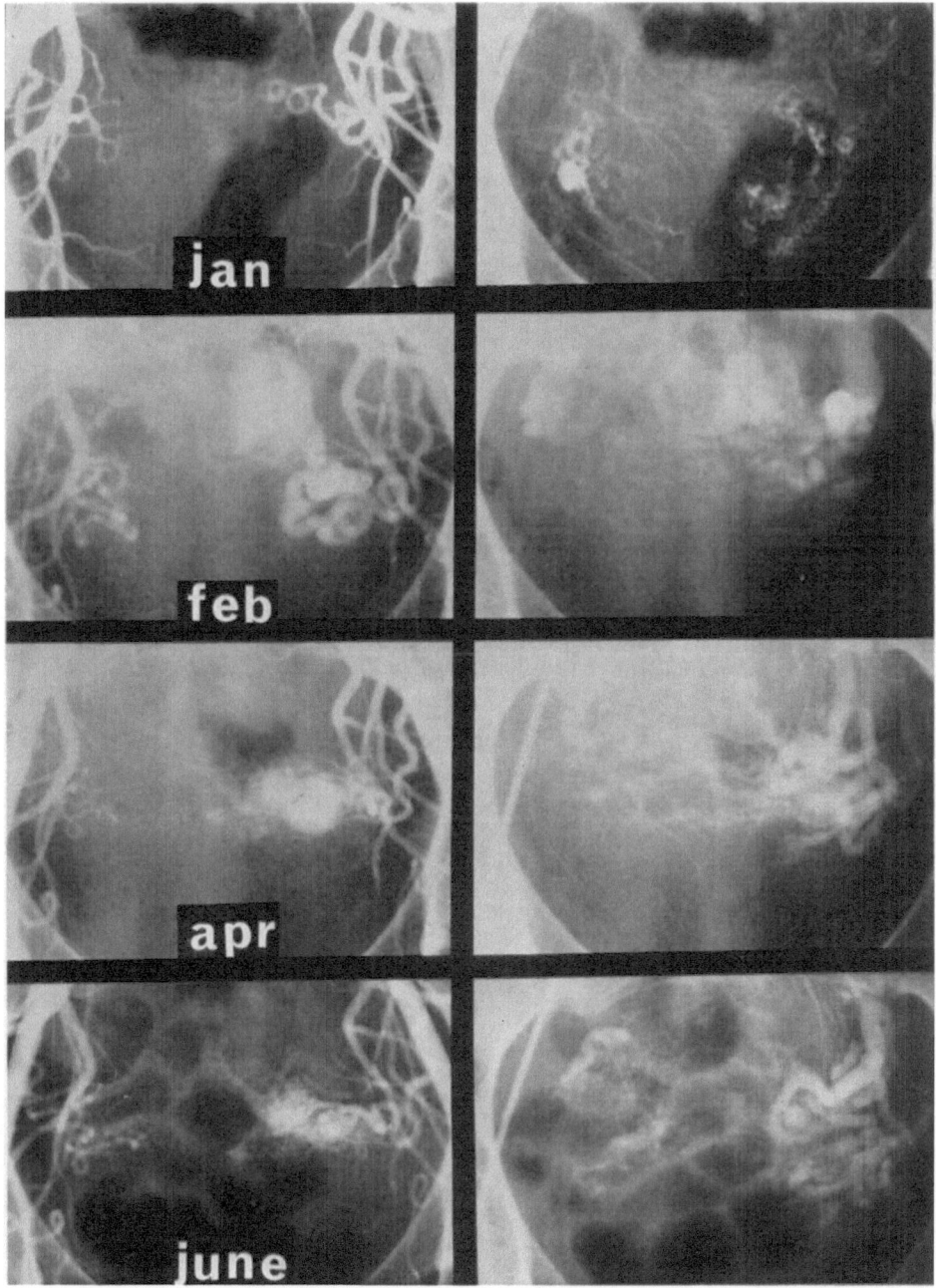

Fig. 3. *January:* Uterine vessels dilated and uterus enlarged but no abnormal vascular spaces. *February:* Uterine vessels greatly enlarged on left and early shunting into ovarian veins. *April:* Uterine vessels smaller but ill defined vascular space persists and irregular draining veins filled by shunting. *June:* Persistent arteriovenous shunting and large plexus of veins apparent in later stages of examination. No irregular vascular spaces. H. C. G. levels normal at time of April and June examinations

cretion levels but negative diagnostic curettages. Pulmonary metastases were present in five of the patients, and the sixth had a small vaginal deposit, the histological appearance of which was typical of choriocarcinoma.

These cases confirm that a normal pelvic angiogram does not necessarily exclude malignant trophoblastic disease elsewhere.

Conclusions

Evidence from the clinical history, the quantitative H.C.G. excretion levels and pelvic angiography provides a safe and reliable method of diagnosing malignant trophoblastic disease.

Following chemotherapy, the pelvic angiogram may return to normal or it may show evidence of persistent arteriovenous fistulae when the initial diagnostic arteriogram demonstrated a shunt. Patients whose tumours become resistant to chemotherapy or recur continue to show abnormal angiographic appearances.

A negative pelvic angiogram does not exclude M.T.D., as deposits elsewhere may persist in the absence of a demonstrable pelvic tumour.

Pelvic angiography provides valuable confirmation of clinical evidence, when combined with H.C.G. excretion studies, of the arrest or remission of malignant trophoblastic tumours in the pelvis.

Acknowledgements

We wish to thank Professor J. B. LAWSON for his help and advice in the preparation of this paper. We also thank our Obstetric and Gynaecological colleagues, Professor G. EDINGTON of the Department of Pathology and Dr. DENNIS BELL of the Department of Radiology for their assistance in this study.

References

ACOSTA-SISON, H., Apparent metastatic chorioepithelioma without demonstrable primary chorionic malignancy in the uterus. *Obstet. and Gynec.* 10, 165—168 (1957).

BAGSHAWE, K. D., *in: Modern Trends in Gynaecology*, London: Butterworth, 1963.

CHAN, D. P. C.: Treatment of chorionepithelioma with methotrexate. *Brit. med. J.* 1962, No 5310, 957—961.

COCKSHOTT, W. P., EVANS, K. T., and HENDRICKSE, J. P., Arteriography of trophoblastic tumors. *Clin. Radiol.* 15, 1—8 (1964).

HENDRICKSE, J. P. d V., COCKSHOTT, W. P., EVANS, K. T. E., and BARTON, C. J., Pelvic angiography in the diagnosis of malignant trophoblastic disease. *New Eng. J. Med.* 271, 859—866 (1964).

HIGHMAN, J. H., and SUTTON, D., Angiography in hydaditiform mole and chorion epithelioma. *Clin. Radiol.* 15, 9—13 (1964).

HOL, R., and INGEBRIGSTEN, R., Experimental arteriovenous fistulae. *Acta radiol. (Stockh.)* 55, 337—349 (1961).

MAIER, H. C., and TAYLOR, H. C., Metastatic chorionepithelioma of the lung treated by lobectomy. *Amer. J. Obstet. Gynec.* 53, 674—677 (1947).

PARK, W. W., and LEES, C. C., Choriocarcinoma. *Arch. Path.* 49, 73—104, 205—241 (1950).

RICHIR, U., QUENUM, C. et CORREA, P., Mole desséqmantes et chorio-épitheliome. *Bull. et Memoires Univ. Dakar* 9, 189—197 (1961).

Diagnosis of Hydatidiform Mole and Related Trophoblastic Diseases

A Further Study of The Galli-Mainini Bioassay Test

Koesoemowardojo, I Wajan Giri, and Moeljono Djojopranoto

Department of Pathology University of Airlangga School of Medicine Surabaja, Indonesia

Introduction

Djojopranota, Lie, and Oei (1963) have reported that the diagnosis of hydatidiform mole can be based upon a positive Galli-Mainini test, e. g. if the patient's urine diluted to 1/400 or higher gives a positive Galli-Mainini result, it can be considered significant. In evaluating the results of the test, however, one must be careful that the hundreth day of pregnancy has not yet passed. Their study utilizing this test on sixty cases of untreated hydatidiform mole gave only 31 positive reactions or 52 per cent.

The aim of this study is to suggest a slight modification of the described method of Djojopranoto *et al.*, 1963 which may be valuable. We wish to propose that the results of the Galli-Mainini tests on the urine of patients with hydatidiform mole which have a titer of less than 1/400, can have significant value if compared with the results of similar tests on urine from normal pregnant women.

Materials and Methods

During a period of $3^1/_2$ years (January 1, 1961 to May 31, 1964) we have studied all cases of hydatitiform mole and related diseases at the Surabaja General Hospital (Table I). These cases had been diagnosed by the examination of microscopic specimens, and the diagnoses were rechecked.

Table I. *All hydatidiform mole and choriocarcinoma cases at the Surabaja General Hospital, during a period of $3^1/_2$ years (1961—1964).*

Hydatidiform moles			Choriocarcinomas		
still benign	with subsequent malignancy	total	non-villous	villous type	total
108	9	117	5	11	16

The investigations of mole were made in patients with "living" hydatidiform mole. In these patients the diagnosis had been made, Galli-Mainini tests were performed before therapy, but the vesicles had not been passed.

We have also studied patients who have had repeated Galli-Mainini tests, to determine whether the result became negative after the first evacuation of mole, or whether the mole developed malignant degeneration.

During a period of $6^1/_2$ years (1958—1964), we have studied all patients with living moles who showed positive Galli-Mainini tests in a dilution of less than 1/400.

Values for the GALLI-MAININI titer during normal pregnancy were determined by repeated examination of urine from 25 women with normal pregnancies who knew the exact date of last menstruation. The GALLI-MAININI test was performed every week for each patient from the last expected menstruation until labor. Tests were done on the first morning urine of the patients, according to methods published previously (DJOJO-PRANOTO et al., 1963).

Results

Titer of living mole. There were 36 patients with living mole who had GALLI-MAININI tests before therapy. The results are tabulated in Table II.

From Table II we can conclude, if the GALLI-MAININI test was positive at a dilution of 1/400 or more, at any time of maturity, the diagnosis of hydatidiform mole or other trophoblastic diseases must be considered seriously (32 cases or 89 per cent). [1]

Follow-up of hydatidiform mole. In 75 cases, follow-up by GALLI-MAININI test was carried out until two or more negative results were attained at intervals of two weeks or more (Table III).

Table II. *Bioassay of urine from 36 cases of living hydatidiform mole (prior to therapy).*

Titer	No. of cases	per cent
1/400	32	89.0
1/200	3	8.33
1/100	1	2.77
less than 1/100	0	—

There were 59 cases (78.6 per cent), in which the GALLI-MAININI test became negative within 4 weeks after the first evacuation of the moles. None of these cases has developed malignant degeneration and all are still benign. Of 16 cases in which the tests remained positive for 6 weeks or more, 7 cases were lost in the follow-up and 9 cases (12 per cent) subsequently developed choriocarcinomas of villous [invasive and/or metastatic mole — Ed] or non-villous type.

Moles with titer less than 1/400 dilution. There were 12 hydatidiform mole cases in which the titers were less than 1/400 during a study of 6^1/$_2$ years. We

[1] These findings are useful for screening purposes, and therefore all suspected amenorrhea patients are screened with this procedure.

Table III. *Time needed to obtain a negative Galli-Manini test of 75 cases, after therapy.*

weeks	No. of cases	per cent	
1	15	20	still benign
2	26	34.6	still benign
3	12	16	still benign
4	6	8	still benign
5	0	—	—
6	1	1.3	subsequent malignancy
7	5	6.6	four cases were lost in follow-up
			one case with subsequent malignancy
8	4	5.3	one case was lost in follow-up
			three cases with subsequent malignancy
9	1	1.3	subsequent malignancy
10	2	2.6	one case was lost in follow-up
			on case with subsequent malignancy
more than 10	3	4	one case was lost in follow-up
			two cases with subsequent malignancy
Total:	75	100	nine cases (twelve per cent), all with subsequent malignancy

compared the titers of these cases with titers of normal pregnancy.

In normal pregnancies, the GALLI-MAININI test is positive within 2 weeks after the last expected menstruation-day or 6 weeks after the first day of the last menses. There is only one case which shows a positive result within one week after the last expected menses or 5 weeks after the first day of the last menses. The tidiform mole (52 per cent) had titers of 1/400 or more, and 20 cases (33.3 per cent) had titers of 1/200. The same figures are respectively 40 per cent and 23 per cent according to CHUN, et al., (1964). But in these two author's papers it was not mentioned whether the moles were still living or not. CHUN et al., (1964), combined moles of group III (vesicles not passed) with moles of group II (ve-

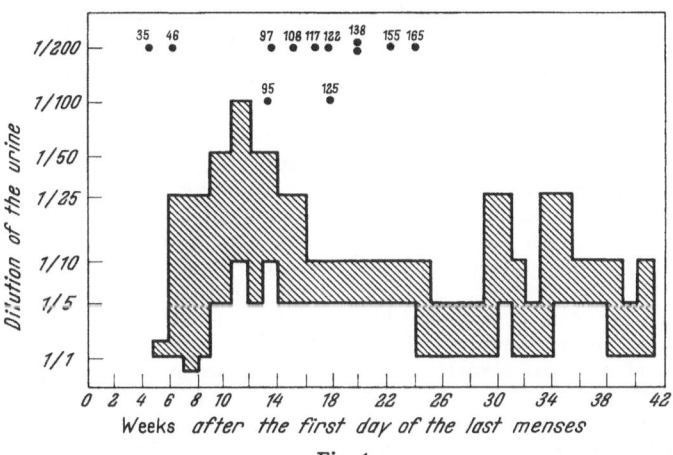

Fig. 1.

titer shows 3 peaks. The highest titer is at the 11th week after the first day of the last menses (1/100). After the 14th week the titer is 1/25 and the plateau level is 1/10 after the 16th week. The other two peaks are at the 30th week and 34th week, each of which are in a dilution of 1/25. (Fig. 1.)

There are ten cases of living mole with a titer of 1/200. Two of these cases occurred at the 35th and 46th day after the first day of the last menses; one case at the 97th day and seven cases at longer than the 100th day.

There are two cases of living mole with titers of 1/100 at the 95th and the 125th day.

Discussion and conclusions

According to DJOJOPRANOTO, LIE and OEI (1963), only 31 patients with hyda-

sicles passed before the investigations were completed). *In the present study, we conclude that a positive GALLI-MAININI test from urine diluted to 1/400 or more, at any time of maturity, indicates the presence of hydatidiform mole or other trophoblastic diseases (32 cases or 89 per cent).*

The HCG (human chorionic gonadotropin hormone) titer in serum compared with morning urine has been found to be very similar. The HCG level in urine appeared to be somewhat proportional to the specific gravity of the urine, and if there was any condition in which the specific gravity of the urine is high, such as in hyperemesis gravidarum, the HCG concentration of the urine may also be high (MISHELL, WIDE and GEMZELL (1963). WIDE (quoted by MISHELL et al.,) has shown that the concentration of the hormone in the first morning urine is similar to that in the 24 hour specimen. Thus it can be concluded that the urine assay has a significant value, although one has to consider that the value given by one laboratory can differ from that of another.

We have observed the size of the uterus in patients with mole and with amenorrhea less than the 100th day to be much larger than the uterus in normal pregnancies, but in those with amenorrhea longer than 100 days, the uterus is about the same size in the normal pregnancies.

Acknowledgments

We would like to express our very grateful thanks to the following for making this study possible: to Dr SOETOMO JOEDOSEPOETRO and Dr. TJOA KIEM LIAN, of Dept. of Obstetrics and Gynecology, University of Airlanga; and to Dr. RUTH A. BOAK and Dr. KELLOGG, visiting Professors at the University of Airlangga, for their helpful criticism and advice in preparation of this manuscript. Also, we should like to acknowledge Mr. KASTARI MERTOWIDJOJO and Miss HARTINI in preparation of this manuscript.

References

ACOSTA-SISON, H., The occurence of malignancy in a repeated hydatidiform mole. *Amer. J. Obstet. Gynec.* 78, 876—877 (1959).

— Chorioadenoma destruens; a report of 41 cases. *Amer. J. Obstet. Gynec.* 80, 176—179 (1960).

ALBERT, A., and BERKSON, J., A clinical bioassay for chorionic gonadotropin. *J. clin. Endocrinol.* 11, 805—820 (1951).

CHUN, D., BRAGA, C., CHOW, C., and LOK, L., Clinical observations on some aspects of hydatidiform moles. *J. Obstet. Gynec. Brit. Cwlth* 71, 180—184 (1964a).

— — — — Treatment of hydatidiform mole. *J. Obstet. Gynaec. Brit. Cwlth* 71, 185—191 (1964b).

DELFS, E., Chorionic gonadotrophin determinations in patients with hydatidiform mole and choriocarcinoma. *Ann. N. Y. Acad. Sci.* 80, 125—139 (1959).

DJOJOPRANOTO, M., LIE, S. L., and OEI, H. H.-K., Biologic pregnancy tests in diagnosis and therapy of hydatidiform mole and choriocarcinoma. *Amer. J. Obstet. Gynec.* 85, 850—855 (1963).

DOUGLAS, G. W., Malignant change in trophoblastic tumors. *Amer. J. Obstet. Gynec.* 84, 884—894 (1962).

HERTIG A. T., and MANSELL, H., Tumors of the female sex organs, part I. Hydatidiform and choriocarcinoma. *In: Atlas of Tumor Pathology*, Sect. IX, Fasc. 33. Armed Forces Institute of Pathology, Washington, 1956.

HOBSON, B. M., Excretion of chorionic gonadotrophin in normal pregancy and in women with hydatidiform mole. *J. Obstet. Gynaec. Brit. Emp.* 52, 354—363 (1955).

HSU, C. T., HUANG, L. C., and CHEN, T. Y., Metastases in benign hydatidiform mole and chorioadenoma destruens. *Amer. J. Obstet. Gynec.* 84, 1412—1424 (1926).

LORAINE, J. A., Clinical Application of Hormone Assay, p. 65—98. Edinburg: Livingstone 1958).

McCARTHY, C., PENNINGTON, G. W., and CRAWFORD W. S., Chorionic gonadotrophin excretion in normal and abnormal pregnancy. *J. Obstet. Gynaec. Brit. Cwlth* 71, 86—91 (1964).

MIDGLEY, A. R., JR., and PIERCE, G. B., JR., Immunohistochemical localization of human chorionic gonadotropin. *J. exp. Med.* 115, 289—294 (1962).

MISHELL, D. R., WIDE, L., and GEMZELL, C. A., Immunologic determination of human chorionic gonadotropin in serum. *J. clin. Endocr.* 23, 125—131 (1963).

NOVAK, F. R., and JONES, G. S., *Novak's Textbook of Gynecology*, ed. 6, p. 612—633. Baltimore: (Williams & Wilkins Co., 1961).

SCHIFFER, M. A., POMERANCE, W., and MACKLES, A., Hydatidiform mole in relation to malignant disease of the trophoblast. *Amer. J. Obstet. Gynec.* 80, 516—531 (1960).

SCOTT, J. S., Choriocarcinoma; observations on the etiology. *Amer. J. Obstet. Gynec.* 83, 185—193 (1962).

WIDE, L.: quoted by Mishell et al.

WYNN, R. M., and DAVIES, J., Ultrastructure of transplanted choriocarcinoma and its endocrine implications. *Amer. J. Obstet. Gynec,* 88, 618—633 (1964).

Comments on the Measurement of HCG
as a Tumor Specific Substance

K. D. BAGSHAWE, M. D., M. R. C. P.,

Charing Cross Hospital Medical School, Fulham Hospital, London W 6, England

The management of cancer therapy generally is handicapped by lack of information about the number of the specific cells we are aiming to destroy. We need tumour specific index substances in order:

a) to establish the diagnosis,

b) to indicate the cellular response to therapeutic agents,

c) to indicate, by their absence in very sensitive systems, complete tumour destruction.

Chorionic gonadotrophin (H. C. G.) is the only tumour specific substance so far usable for this purpose. As such it is unique. It is regrettable that it is still being measured by a wide variety of methods which originated as qualitative tests for pregnancy and which are not suitable as quantitative assays. (BAGSHAWE and WILDE, 1965).

HCG has been assayed in almost every animal in laboratory captivity. The answers obtained from assays performed without the inclusion of reference standards and expressed in animal units are not open to strict quantitative interpretation. It is useful to consider what properties an ideal tumour index substance would have so that we know what to look for — and then we can see how close we can get to this with HCG (Table I).

Our objectives in trying to get better methods for the measurement of HCG can be stated in the order of priority we have adopted in our laboratory.

1. Sensitivity adequate to detect full range of normal values of luteinizing hormone excretion.

2. Precision, adequate to ensure that the changes seen, are not due to variation in the assay system but are due to changes in tumour metabolism.

3. To be able to distinguish HCG from LH. This will give a zero base line and allow us to employ the maximum sensitivity we can achieve.

4. To determine the synthesis rate or secretion rate of HCG.

Immunologic methods are not necessarily superior to biological methods except insofar as they generally permit a wide range of possible values to be covered in a single assay with reasonable cost in time and money. During the past 4 years we have employed biological assays against sub-standards of the International Reference Preparation of HCG as a research tool to develop new assay methods. We have rejected latex agglutination and complement fixation as these methods are unsuitable for various reasons. Haemagglutination inhibition using

Table I. *A comparison of the properties of chorionic gonadotrophin with those of an ideal tumour specific index substance.*

Ideal tumour index substance	Chorionic gonadotrophin (HCG)
1. Produced specifically by the tumour cells and no other.	1. Yes. But HGG cross-reacts with luteinizing hormone (LH) in both biological and immunological systems.
2. One cell produces enough to be detected.	2. No. But potential sensitivity of new methods for HCG is very great.
3. Chemically stable and not rapidly metabolised.	3. Relatively stable in urine. Half life in body fluids not yet determined.
4. High renal clearance so that excretion is close to synthesis rate or secretion rate of the hormone.	4. No. Approximately 1 ml./min.
5. If low renal rate of clearance, synthesis rate determinable by other methods.	5. Probably.
6. Measureable by simple methods. Capable of automation.	6. Probably.

pyruvic aldehyde fixation of red cells as described by Ling (1960) and HCG labelling as described by Butt, Crooke and Cunningham (1961) has proved satisfactory in many respects. The sensitivity of this method is about 1 IU/ml. so that concentration of the hormone in the urine is necessary in order to detect normal levels of gonadotrophin production.

To get closer to making HCG an ideal index substance we have developed a radioimmunoassay (Bagshawe, Wilde and Orr 1966).

This is basically an immuno-precipitation method. When HCG and rabbit anti-HCG sera are allowed to react under suitable conditions and in high concentration, a visible precipitate is formed. When they are mixed in the low concentration necessary to achieve a highly sensitive assay, the antigen-antibody complexes formed, remain in solution. They may be precipitated, however, by the addition of an antiserum to rabbit gamma-globulin. The fine precipitate formed can be filtered off by passing through an 'Oxoid' milli-

pore membrane. When HCG—I^{131} is included in the system the radioactivity recovered on the membrane is related to the concentration of unlabelled HCG in the system.

The specificity of the test is determined by the purity of the labelled protein. Any pure antigenic substance originating specifically in the tumour would be suitable for this purpose but a biologically active protein such as HCG can be purified more readily perhaps because it is readily followed through the separation procedures. The HCG we have used in this procedure, prepared in my laboratory by Dr. C. Wilde, assays between 10,000 and 30,000 IU/mg.

The sensitivity now obtained is 0.007 IU HCG/ml. which is roughly equivalent to 7 IU HCG/L. urine without concentration. The method works with blood; it does not distinguish between LH and HCG. It can be semiautomated. We hope it will enable us to determine the secretion rate of HCG and thus help us to make full use of this very important substance.

Dr. HERTZ referred to the need to keep urine collected for assay at low temperature. This may be the case for mouse bioassays but with immunoassays, chemical bacteriostatics such as sodium azide can be used and are more convenient especially where transportation of the urine is unavoidable.

References

BAGSHAWE, K. D., and WILDE, C. E., Some aspects of the excretion of gonadotrophic hormones by patients with trophoblastic tumours. *J. Obstet. Gynaec. Brit. Cwlth* **72**, 59—64 (1965).

BAGSHAWE, K. D., WILDE, C. E., and ORR, A. H., Radioimmunoassay for human chorionic gonadotrophin and luteinizing hormone. Lancet I, 1118 (1966).

BUTT, W. R., CROOKE, A. C., and CUNNINGHAM, F. J., Studies on human urinary and pituitary gonadotrophins. *Biochem. J.* **81**, 596—605 (1961).

LING, N. R., The attachment of proteins to cells tanned with pyruvic aldehyde. *Biochem. J.* **72**, 12P (1960).

WILDE, C. E., ORR, A. H., HILARY, and BAGSHAWE, K. D., Radioimmunoassay for human chorionic gonadotrophin. *Nature (Lond.)* **205**, 191—192 (1965).

Urinary Estrogen Excretion in Chorionic Tumor Patients

Kohachiro Koga, M. D., and Kozuo Maeda, M. D.

Department of Obstetrics and Gynecology, Faculty of Medicine
Kyushu University, Fukuoka, Japan

Estrogen levels on 24 hour urines were determined by Brown's method in 21 patients with hydatidiform mole, 9 normal pregnant women and 7 normal menstruating women.

The mean total estrogen values were 291.0 µg in patients with hydatidiform mole, 377.4 µg in pregnant women in their first trimester and 46.2 µg in normal menstruating women in the luteal phase.

The corresponding mean estriol values were 27.9 µg in hydatidiform mole patients, 193.1 µg in normal pregnancies and 29.2 µg in normal menstruating women. Thus despite elevated total estrogen excretion the mean estriol level in women with hydatidiform mole was normal. The estradiol values, however, were higher in women with hydatidiform mole than in normal pregnancy or in the luteal phase of the menstrual cycle.

These results indicate disturbance of estrogen metabolism in hydatidiform mole and suggest the usefulness of this procedure in differentiating hydatidiform mole from normal pregnancy.

Total estrogen levels were determined in two patients with choriocarcinoma prior to and after total hysterectomy and salpingo-oophorectomy. The total estrogen excretion in the first patient was 113 µg prior to and 35.1 µg 7 days after surgery. The level increased again to 126 µg when pulmonary metastases appeared. In the second woman the estrogen level was 87.9 µg prior to surgery and 82.0 µg when pulmonary metastases appeared post-operatively. These results support the interpretation that estrogens are produced by choriocarcinomatous tissue.

Quantitative Human Chorionic Gonadotropin Immunoassay

M. M. HRESHCHYSHYN and N. R. ROSE

Assoc. Prof. Obstetrics and Gynecology, State University of New York at Buffalo; and Asociate Cancer Research Gynecologist, Roswell Park Memorial Institute, Buffalo, New York.
Associate Professor, Department of Bacteriology and Immunology, State University of New York at Buffalo, School of Medicine, Buffalo, New York

The quantitative bioassay technique for human chorionic gonadotropin (HCG) discussed by Dr. ROY HERTZ, is a sensitive, accurate and well tested method. We have employed it in our clinic for the past seven years. It is, however, a procedure which is expensive, time consuming and not always adaptable to clinics with little or no laboratory facilities. On the other hand, the immunologic techniques now commonly employed for diagnosis of pregnancy, take little time and are relatively inexpensive. When performed on non-processed urine, however, they are not sensitive enough for quantitative gonadotropin assay.

In an attempt to combine the desirable aspects of both methods, we have performed immunoassays on urine concentrates which were also titered in the bioassay system[1]. The results of the two procedures were compared.

Procedure. An aliquot of a 24 hour urine specimen, not less than 400 cc, was processed by a modified ALBERT's tech-nique. The sample was adjusted to pH 4.5 with glacial acetic acid. Twenty grams of kaolin were added and the suspension was stirred for one minute. The suspension was then filtered with suction through a 15 cm BUCHNER funnel with one sheet each of Whatman paper numbers 40 and 50. The resulting kaolin pack was then rinsed with two liters of tap water to which 1 cc glacial acetic acid was added. For elution from the kaolin, 100 ml of 2N ammonium hydroxide was run through the pack twice, followed by 50 ml of distilled water. The eluate was adjusted to pH 5.0 with glacial acetic acid and precipitated with 300 ml of acetone. Following refrigeration at 5° C for at least 30 minutes, the resulting suspension was centrifuged at 350 G for 15 minutes. The supernatant was poured off and the sediment suspended in 15 ml of distilled water and stored at 5° C. The recovery of added HCG with this procedure in our laboratory has been approximately 80 per cent.

For bioassay, white Swiss mice 15 to 21 days old with body weights of 6 to 12 grams were used. Urine concentrate in serial dilutions was injected into three mice per dilution, each mouse receiving

---

[1] The urines were collected from female patients who were pregnant and who had trophoblastic growths, active or in remission, and from male patients with testicular tumors.

0.5 ml daily for three days. The mice were sacrificed on the fourth day and the uteri were weighed. If two out of three mice doubled the weight of the uterus as compared with the control, the result was called positive. Lesser but definite weight increase (more than 50% average weight increase) was called borderline positive or plus-minus. The results were expressed in mouse uterine units (m. u. u.).

For immunoassay, materials from Wampole Laboratories' Urinary Chorionic Gonadotropin (UCG) test[2] were used. Serial 1:2 dilutions of the urine concentrate were made in physiologic saline. 0.25 ml of these dilutions were added to 0.25 ml of antiserum. 0.04 ml of formalinized human chorionic gonadotropin-coated sheep erythrocytes were added and tubes were agitated. The results were compared with the diluent control in 2 hours. Gonadotropin present in the urine reacted with the antisera, thus blocking the expected reaction with the sensitized red cells. One International Unit in 1.0 ml of saline (0.25 I. U. in the 0.25 ml used in the test) is necessary to inhibit the reaction.

In the immunoassay, however, the presence of other urine constituents in the lower dilutions increases the sensitivity.

The comparison of results on a logarithmic scale is shown in the graph. There is a good correlation of the values in urine specimens containing more than 200 mouse uterine units or 60 I. U./15 ml concentrate. This attests to the usefulness of the quantitative immunoassay procedure as described for clinical purposes in patients with trophoblastic neoplasia.

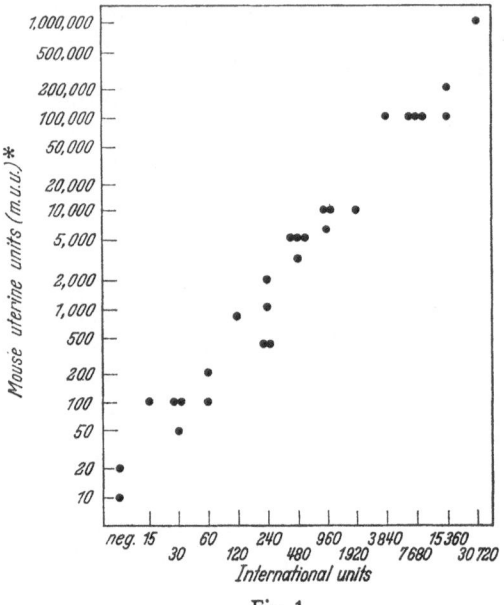

Fig. 1

[2] Wampole Laboratories, 35 Commerce Road, Stamford, Connecticut.

Synopsis of Discussion IV

Dr. Holland raised the question whether poor prognosis in individuals with exceptionally high titers represented a type of tumor with greater derepression of normal trophoblastic function. Dr. Hertz stated his view that the gonadotropin titer is a reflection of the amount of biologically active tumor in the body. His experience with patients and with assays in chorionic tumor tissue growing in hamsters indicated that there was a fairly uniform range of biological potency of tumors and of tumor homo-genates. He chose to interpret gonadotropin titer roughly as indicating extent of disease rather than malignancy of the cell type. Dr. Holland counseled against picking an arbitrary point in time (4 months) and calculating prognosis before and after. Rather, since time is only an indirect parameter by which one measures disease effects on the patient, an analysis of these effects and of tumor size might be more meaningful. Dr. Hertz indicated that the only objective factor he could find in analysis of histories and in clinical observations was time, and that no specific biochemical indicator of effects on the host was available.

Dr. HEDNRICKSE reported his experience in 46 of 61 patients with trophoblastic neoplasms, the remaining 15 being currently under treatment. 43 of the 46 had metastasis and 29 of these are in complete remission (67 %). The remaining 3 non-metastatic patients all sustained complete remission. Among those with metastases, surgery and chemotherapy were employed in some (64 % in remission) and chemotherapy alone in the remainder (68 %). Methotrexate resistance was encountered four times. He had abandoned arbitrary dosage of methotrexate and was now giving methotrexate and 6-mercaptopurine adjusted according to body weight.

Dr. BAGSHAWE indicated, in response to questioning, that he was reluctant to infuse methotrexate as high as the ovarian supply, in an attempt to saturate the entire circulation of a trophoblastic neoplasm. He preferred to lodge his catheter immediately above the bifurcation because the risks of high drug concentration to the kidney and to the renal and inferior mesenteric vessels would attend attempts at ovarian arterial drug administration. Furthermore, in his regimen, oral 6-mercaptopurine and/or the infused methotrexate produced some leukopenia, implying a systemic effect.

Dr. CHAN noted that it had been observed in Singapore that the latent period between hydatidiform mole and the appearance of invasive or metastatic mole was shorter than that between hydatidiform mole and choriocarcinoma. Thus the higher mortality which occurs in cases recrudescent long after the appearance of mole may be a manifestation of a group histologically and dynamically more serious than patients found earlier. Dr. FINKELSTEIN commented on prolonged regressions with absent gonadotropin and subsequent recrudescence and death. He is aware of a perfectly normal pregnancy with normal delivery in which the pregnancy test was completely negative until 6 months of gestation in several reliable laboratories. Thus, even normal placenta sometimes might lose its capacity to secrete gonodotropin.

Chemotherapy of Chorionic Tumors

NAOTAKA ISHIZUKA, M. D.

*Professor of Obstetrics and Gynecology, Nagoya University School of Medicine,
Nagoya, Japan*

I want to present here the results of chemotherapy and other treatments of chorionic tumors in our clinic during a period of 13 years from 1950 to 1963. These cases were histologically classified under the diagnoses of chorionepithelioma [choriocarcinoma-Ed] and destructive mole [invasive mole-Ed] according to Ewing and Novak's criteria.

Table I shows the number of cases of chorionic tumors classified. We have called an "undetermined case" a patient in whom we were unable to find chorionic tissue in the uterus and the diagnosis was made on pulmonary lesions.

Table II shows the prognosis of the total cases summarized. Of 37 cases of chorionepithelioma, 7 survived more than one year. Thirty other cases died. Of destructive mole, 58 of 63 cases survived for more than one year. Five other cases died.

There were 49 patients treated with chemotherapeutic agents out of the 101 cases mentioned above (Table III). As a rational approach it is recommended that patients with evidence of metastasis be put on chemotherapeutic evaluation. Still, it seems essential to perform a radical operation in treating chorionepithelioma. Chemotherapy is a necessary procedure

Table I. *Numbers of cases of chorionic tumors*

Classification	Number of cases
Chorionepithelioma	37
Destructive Mole	63
Undetermined	1
Total	101

Table II. *Prognosis*

Classification	Survived for			Died
	Less than 2 years (over one year)	More than 2 years	Total	
Chorionepithelioma	2	5	7 (19%)	30 (81%)
Destructive Mole	8	50	58 (92%)	5 (8%)
Undetermined	0	1	1	0
Total	10	56	66 (65%)	35 (35%)

to fill a gap left uncovered. Out of 49 cases 23 were combined with operation, 24 with operation and other treatments and the remaining 2 were treated by chemotherapy alone.

Table IV shows the varieties of chemotherapeutic agents administered. Nitromin was mostly used in this study because it was produced in the earlier stage of chemotherapy in our country.

Table V shows the relation between the site of metastasis and the prognosis of chemotherapeutic cases. In this table, living patients are shown above and fatal cases below the middle dividing line. The site of metastasis is divided into two groups: "adjacent" means parametrium, vagina and vulva; "distant" means lung, brain and so on. "Unknown" means the

case in which I could not find the focus of metastasis in spite of a positive pregnancy test.

Table III. *Combination of treatments*

Cases of chemotherapy	49
Combined with operation	23
Combined with operation and other treatments	24
Chemotherapy alone	2

One case of chorionepithelioma was cured by chemotherapy despite evident pulmonary metastasis. Twenty-six other cases all died of distant metastasis. On the other hand, as to destructive mole, 19 out of 21 cases were cured. Of the 19 cured cases, 9 cases showed evidence of

Table IV. *Varieties of chemotherapeutic agents administered*

Chemotherapeutic Agents	Numbers of Cases	Administration		
		Method	Daily Dose (mg)	Total Dose (mg)
Nitrogen Mustard N-oxide (Nitromin)	36	intravenous	25—50	75—2875
Amethopterin (Methotrexate)	11	oral	5—25	25—1155
Mitomycin C	8	intravenous	2—4	26—60
Cyclophosphamide (Endoxan)	4	intravenous	50—100	2200—5900
8-Azaguanin (Azan)	3	intramuscular	40	400
Chromomycin A_3 (Toyomycin)	2	intravenous	0.5	5—7.5
Thiotepa (Tespamin)	1	intramuscular	5	150
Sarkomycin	1	intravenous	1000	5000
Nitrogen Mustard	1	intravenous	5	10

Table V. *The relation between the site of metastasis and prognosis of chemotherapeutic cases*

	Metastasis		Chorionepithelioma		Destructive mole		Undetermined	
Survived 21 (43%)	positive	distant	1	1	9	19	1	1
		adjacent	0	(4%)	5	(90%)	0	
		unknown	0		3		0	
	negative		0		2		0	
Died 28 (57%)	positive	distant	26	26	1	2	0	0
		adjacent	0	(96%)	1	(10%)	0	
		unknown	0		0		0	
	negative		0		0		0	
Total 49 (100%)				27 (100%)		21 (100%)		1

obvious pulmonary metastasis. One of the two fatal cases died of sepsis and the other, diagnosed destructive mole according to Novak's histological criteria, of brain metastasis.

These data are the results of therapy performed up to the summer of 1964. Ever since, we have been studying the value of methotrexate for metastatic chorionic tumors. We have the impression that this agent may possess, to some extent, a better effect. Measurement of gonadotropin titre with serological test procedures is being used to follow the clinical course.

A clarification of histological characteristics of the primary lesion will lead to a perspective of the subsequent chemotherapy. It is not rare that destructive mole is accompanied by metastasis. Fortunately, such metastasis has promise of a high cure rate by chemotherapeutic agents. In treating metastatic cases of chorionepithelioma, chemotherapy does not seem so effective, but is by no means hopeless. Nine cases of choriocarcinoma showed a temporary remission and one case had a permanent cure. I would like to hope that more effective and harmless agents will appear in the near future.

The Use of 6-Mercaptopurine with Methotrexate in the Treatment of Trophoblastic Tumors

K. D. Bagshawe, M.D., M.R.C.P.,

Charing Cross Hospital Medical School, Fulham Hospital, London, W. 6, England

Preliminary considerations

The objectives of a therapeutic attack on trophoblastic tumours can be defined in order of priority. The first is total and permanent elimination of the tumour with the least possible risk to the life of the patient. Subsidiary objectives are the preservation of function of the affected organs, the prevention of infection and its consequences during treatment, the avoidance of drug toxicity and a short period of hospitalisation.

The therapy of trophoblastic tumours is closely interwoven with the diagnostic problem and it is therefore necessary to consider what is implied by our concept of "indications for treatment". This concept contains two components. One is the threat to life or health which is implicit in the patient's disease pattern. The other is the risk inherent in the therapy. The clinician's initial task is therefore to assess the threat of the particular disease pattern. This threat may be immediate or ultimate.

The immediate threat to life constitutes an indication for specific treatment, provided there is corroborative evidence of trophoblastic disease.

The immediate threats encountered in this series have been severe uterine and vaginal haemorrhage, uterine perforation, embolic pulmonary hypertension and evidence of intracranial metastases.

An assessment of the ultimate or non-immediate threat is necessarily based on all the information which can be obtained. Key features are: (1) the interval since the antecedent pregnancy; (2) the nature of that pregnancy; (3) the location and the extent of metastases; (4) precise quantitative measurements (in International Units) of H.C.G. excretion and the inclination of the H.C.G. excretion, i.e. whether increasing, constant, or decreasing; (Bagshawe and Wilde, 1965, Wilde *et al*, 1965). (5) The findings on pelvic arteriography and (6) the histological findings.

These criteria also form a basis for clinical classification. But clearly it is the overall pattern of disease in which the threat to life must be recognized, and not the label conferred by this classification or any other.

When the disease pattern in a patient predicts a fatal course, almost any risks due to treatment may have to be accepted, but as the certainty of a fatal outcome diminishes so the importance of the risk inherent in treatment increases. Obiously, as treatment is made safer, so the threshold for treatment may be lowered and less advanced disease treated, with the benefits this is likely to bring.

It is appropriate to consider at this point whether hysterectomy should be performed in order to get histological evidence. Arguments against this practice are: (1) it may fail to produce evidence, (2) the evidence it may provide may be misleading, (3) it may prejudice the course of the disease and (4) it precludes further pregnancy.

The place of hysterectomy as a therapeutic procedure has also to be assessed. It is difficult to justify hysterectomy where extra-uterine disease already exists, except when there is uterine perforation. Where there is no extra-uterine disease and where the woman has children, hysterectomy offers some prospect of success with relatively small risks. However, evidence that hysterectomy may prejudice the response to drugs will be given later. If this is confirmed, hysterectomy would be strongly contra-indicated, at least until such time as our therapeutic equipment is adequate to overcome the disadvantages which hysterectomy might confer.

The chemotherapy of a tumour is of course, a far more complex affair than the simple administration of this or that agent, and the clinicians' interpretation of certain characteristic features of trophoblastic tumours must influence techniques. Trophoblast penetrates the pelvic venous circulation and fragments of this tissue break away and impact on the arterial side of the pulmonary circulation. (SCHMORL, 1904, DOUGLAS et al., 1959, BAGSHAWE and BROOKS, 1959). Studies have shown that more than 20% of the right ventricular output may be diverted through pulmonary arterio-venous shunts in these patients. (BAGSHAWE and NOBLE, 1966.) Evidence of spontaneous tumour embolization to the lungs has been present in about one quarter of the patients in this series, but embolic phenomena have been an almost invariable accompaniment of treatment.

Drug toxicity

Since we know, that at least initially, the trophoblastic cells are more sensitive than the normal cells to the agents used, it is theoretically possible to achieve a therapeutic effect without toxicity even with systemic therapy. In practice this is not achieved, although in some patients total tumour destruction can be achieved with remarkably little toxicity. Toxicity can be avoided of course, by reducing the drug concentrations, or the duration of each course of drugs, but the danger is, that if total tumour destruction is not obtained within a short time, the development of drug resistance is favoured. Unfortunately there is no way of telling at the outset which tumours are highly sensitive and which are not.

The average course of treatment by our regimen reduces the white cell count to 1500 to 2000 per cu. mm. but where there is evidence of more than average tumor resistance, W.B.C. counts of less than 500 W.B.C. per cu. mm. may follow the regimen then adopted.

Toxicity has many aspects and each requires individual attention. At modest degrees of leukopenia, stomatitis and proctitis are the only common toxic manifestations, but infection is an ever present hazard. Until MARCH, 1964, the patients in this series were nursed in open 30-bed general medical wards and despite a helpful and detailed bacteriological routine, infection was not infrequent. Since MARCH, 1964, the patients have been nursed in an ultra-clean isolation unit which was specially designed for patients with chorionepithelioma (BAGSHAWE, 1964). Our bacteriological routine generally allows us to predict the likely agents where an infection occurs and to use the appropriate antibiotics without the usual delay of 48 hours for antibiotic tests.

One other aspect which requires anticipation is the loss of gut mucosal surface. We have noticed that patients with extensive mucosal loss absorb otherwise poorly absorbed substances. Under these conditions endotoxin shock is also liable to occur, and can be fatal. The bacterial flora may be reduced with suitable antibiotics, provided they are given sufficiently far ahead.

Drug resistance and results

The prevention of drug resistance and overcoming established drug resistance have been major considerations in this study. At the outset, a favourable impression was formed of the combination of methotrexate with 6-mercaptopurine in the treatment of choriocarcinoma. The use of either agent alone has been avoided whenever possible. The value of 6-mercaptopurine given by itself has therefore not been assessed in this study, except for a single course of treatment given to one patient. (BAGSHAWE, 1962). This produced a favourable response as judged by the effect on gonadotrophin excretion. SUNG HUNG CHAO et al. (1963), have used 6-mercaptopurine by itself, in a well documented series of trophoblastic tumours, and the results obtained were very similar to those obtained with methotrexate alone.

6-mercaptopurine has been used in various combinations with folic acid antagonists in the treatment of acute leukaemias in numerous studies. Some authors have not found the combination advantageous, but others have. These studies have been reviewed by SAMPEY, (1961).

WOODLIFF, (1963), has studied the sensitivity of mouse leukaemic cells by measuring their oxygen uptake in Warburg apparatus. He used 3 strains of cell and found good correlation between the effect on the disease in vivo and the effect on oxygen consumption in vitro. Methotrexate inhibited the oxygen uptake of a methotrexate sensitive strain of cells and also of a strain of cells resistant to 6-mercaptopurine. 6-mercaptopurine inhibited the oxygen uptake of 6-mercaptopurine sensitive cells, but not of methotrexate resistant cells.

The overall figures of this series (Table I) show that of 81 patients referred for treatment 56 have been treated with chemotherapy, and 11 of these are still under treatment.

The basic regimen consists of methotrexate 25 mg./day divided in 5 doses per day, with courses of 3—6 days duration. The exact duration is determined on the 3rd, 4th and 5th days. Whenever methotrexate is given, 6-mercaptopurine is also given, and the dosage has varied between 200 and 700 mg./day. (BAGSHAWE and McDONALD, 1960; BAGSHAWE, 1963). Recently the smaller doses of 6-mercaptopurine have generally been used.

Whenever possible, treatment has been continued for 6—8 weeks after normal gonadotrophin excretion levels have been obtained.

Amongst 41 patients treated with methotrexate and 6-mercaptopurine from the beginning there have been 4 instances of drug resistance and two of these subsequently remitted with other measures. Four patients started treatment at other hospitals with methotrexate alone and 2 of these subsequently became resistant to methotrexate and 6-mercaptopurine in combination.

Of the 45 patients treated, 6 have died and the remainder are in complete remission (Table 2). Three patients have residual defects due to structural damage caused by the disease, or due to complications of therapy. The longest remission

Table I. *Trophoblastic tumors*

Patients referred or seen with alleged trophoblastic disease:	*Total*	*81*
No evidence of trophoblastic disease	1	
Treated, with non-standard regime (Surgery ± methotrexate ± Deep x-ray)	10	
Trophoblastic disease which regressed spontaneously (includes 2 with pulmonary metastases)	11	
Died within 4 days of admission from advanced disease	3	25
Treated with methotrexate and 6-mercaptopurine		
(a) Completed treatment. Complete remissions	39	
(b) Died	6	
(c) Currently under treatment	11	*56*
		81

Analysis of treated cases (a, b above)		Total 45	Died 6	
Preceding pregnancy	Molar	26	4	
	Non-molar	19	2	
Race	European	39	3	
	African	5	3	
	Anglo-Chinese	1	0	
Histology	Choriocarcinoma	24	5	
	Invasive Mole	3	0	
	Undetermined	18	1	
Metastases	Brain or Retina	9	4	
	Lung-Parenchymal	34	5	
	Intravascular only	6	0	
	None recognized	5	1	
Interval from onset	0—4 months	16	1	(R)
of symptoms (or from	5—8 months	11	3	(R, S, S)
evacuation of mole)	9—12 months	9	0	
to start of chemotherapy	13—24 months	6	1	(R)
(Mean 8.2 months).	24+ months	3	1	(S)
Systemic Chemotherapy only				
With MTX and 6-MP throughout		31	4	
Initially with MTX alone		4	2	
Infusion therapy		10	0	
Hysterectomized patients		16	5	
Non-hysterectomized patients		29	1	

R = Drug Resistant; S = Drug Sensitive

is 6 years, the most recent two months, and the mean is in excess of 2 years.

There have been no late relapses, but 4 patients have shown rising titres within two months of discontinuing treatment, and after further treatment, 3 of these have had remissions, which have been sustained. All the 6 failures occurred in the first 20 treated cases, and there have been no failures subsequently, but we are not optimistic enough to suppose that a 100% recovery rate can be maintained. Six patients have had seven normal pregnancies subsequent to therapy, and there have been no foetal abnormalities or further molar pregnancies so far (DUMOULIN and BAGSHAWE, 1963).

In particular patients, this regimen has been modified substantially. For instance, patients with intracranial metastases may develop intracranial haemorrhage if rapid necrosis occurs. We have therefore used a low dosage regimen in such patients (5 mg. methotrexate and 100 mg. of 6-mercaptopurine twice daily), and this has been discontinued when toxicity appears.

It is possible that this low dosage regimen increases the risk of drug resistance developing, but this risk may be of a lower order than that of intracranial haemorrhage.

Chlorambucil, vinblastine, nitrogen mustard, actinomycin D, ethoglucid, parahydroxypropiophenone and immunotherapy were used without permanent benefit in the drug resistant patients, but because of the small number of such patients, a negative result does not necessarily indicate that these agents are valueless. Our main effort continues to be directed towards maintaining the initial sensitivity of the tumour to the folic acid and purine antagonists.

Until recently it did not seem possible to explain the action of methotrexate solely on the basis of its affinity for folic reductase enzymes, or of resistance to it, solely on the basis of increased folic reductase synthesis. The success of combined metabolite-antimetabolite infusion therapy was inconsistent with this concept, as was BURCHENAL's demonstration (1951) of a competitive action between methotrexate and folinic acid. But WERKHEISER's study (1963) of the concentration dynamics of the folate and anti-folate compounds, may restore its plausibility. Serveral other possible explanations of drug resistance have been identified. JACOBSON (1961) has shown that some cells can inactivate methotrexate possibly by terminal ring closure. He has also suggested that some tumour cells, like some bacteria, can synthesize folate compounds from suitable precursors, and this raises the possibility of feeding such cells with antagonistically configurated precursors. Alternatively, cells might develop folate pathways which are not blocked by methotrexate, or their D.N.A. synthesis might proceed in the absence of folate activity. Fortunately there is no evidence so far to suggest that either of these last two mechanisms are operative.

On the basis of these and other theoretical considerations we have modified our therapeutic regimen. For the last 27 months all our patients on systemic therapy have been kept on a diet of low folic acid content, (about 25 μg/day). During a 2-year period we had only one instance of drug resistance, but in the past three months we have encountered 3 further instances. Pyrimethamine has been added to the regimen of these patients but it is too early to assess its value. In addition we are experimenting with methods aimed at depressing the synthesis of dihydrofolic reductase. A strong theoretical case can be made for this approach and the results so far obtained appear both interesting and encouraging. Three of the four patients so treated now have normal gonadotrophin values but continue under treatment. If substantiated, this method of therapy may have far reaching consequences on the application of antimetabolite therapy in general.

Analysis of our results has shown that patients who have undergone hysterectomy have generally responded less readily to chemotherapy than those who have not. Hysterectomized subjects have more commonly shown drug resistance. Five of the six deaths have been in the 16 hysterectomized patients and only one in the 29 non-hysterectomized patients but the numbers involved are too small for this to be regarded as conclusive.

Infusion therapy

The occurence of pregnancies in successfully treated patients emphasized the anomalous situation which has arisen. If a patient is not diagnosed till distant metastases have developed, hysterectomy is not usually carried out. Such patients, after successful treatment with chemotherapy, can have normal children. If, however, diagnosis is established early in the disease, hysterectomy may be carried out and in a sense the patient is penalized for early diagnosis. This is especially the case when chemotherapy is necessary after hysterectomy has been done. Even so there is a natural reluctance to subject patients to systemic chemotherapy if it can possibly be avoided.

We have therefore treated patients who have evidence of pelvic tumours, but no evidence of extra pelvic metastases, by an infusion technique. This has been described in some detail elsewhere, (Bagshawe and Wilde 1964). A polytetrafluoroethylene catheter of about 1 mm. internal bore is introduced percutaneously in the femoral artery, and advanced to a point just above the bifurcation of the aorta. Through this, methotrexate is infused at a constant rate of 25 mg./day. The infusions have been continued for periods of up to 20 days, but they are usually interrupted after 10 days, and the catheter is kept patent with saline. The infusion has then been continued for a further period. During the methotrexate infusion, 6-mercaptopurine has been given 200 mg./day, by mouth, and folinic acid has been given intramuscularly at a rate of 9—15 mg./day.

The same catheter may remain in situ for 6—8 weeks, but earlier replacement may be needed if the patient has evidence of local or systemic infection. During the infusion, pulmonary embolism occurs as it does with systemic therapy. This is considered to result from intravascular necrosis of tumour in pelvic veins. The possibility of growth of such tumour fragments in the lungs is a risk, and has occurred in at least one patient. If extra pelvic growth is established, systemic chemotherapy may be indicated, but the amount of systemic therapy required so far has always been small.

Ten patients treated in this way have not developed significant alopecia or stomatitis. If the infusion is prolonged, leucopenia occurs. Even when systemic therapy is subsequently necessary, the patients are at least spared a substantial part of the toxic effects.

But this is a method which should be used only by those already experienced in chemotherapy and in the technical problems of infusion therapy.

Many difficulties in the management of trophoblastic tumours remain to be overcome, but sufficient progress has been made to let us define and approach the problems with precision and clear purpose.

References

Bagshawe, K. D., Treatment of choriocarcinoma with a combination of cytotoxic drugs. *Brit. med. J.* 1960 II, 426—431.
— The chemotherapy of chorionepithelima. In: *Modern Trends in Gynecology*, ed. Kellar, R. J., London: Butterworth, 1962.
— Trophoblastic tumours. Chemotherapy and developments. *Brit. med. J.* 1963 II, 1303—1307.

Bagshawe, K. D., Ultra-clean ward for cancer chemotherapy. *Brit. med. J.* 1964 II, 871—872.
— and Brooks, W. D. W., Subacute pulmonary hypertension due to chorionepithelioma. *Lancet* 1959 I, 653—658.
— and Noble, M. I. M., Cardio-respiratory aspects of trophoblastic tumors. *Quart. J. Med.* 35, 39—54 (1966).

BAGSHAWE, K. D., and WILDE, C. E., Infusion therapy for pelvic trophoblastic tumours. *J. Obstet Gynec. Brit. Cwlth* 71, 565—570 (1964).

— — Some aspects of the excretion of gonadotrophic hormones by patients with trophoblastic tumours. *J. Obstet. Gynec. Brit. Cwlth* 72, 59—64 (1965).

BURCHENAL, J. H., and BABCOCK, G. M., Prevention of toxicity of massive doses of A-methopterin by citrovorum factor. *Proc. Soc exp. Biol (N. Y.)* 76, 382—384 (1951).

DOUGLAS, G. W., THOMAS, L., CARR, M., CULLIN, N. M., and MORRIS, R., Trophoblast in the circulating blood during pregnancy. *Amer. J. Obstet Gynec.* 78, 960—973 (1959).

DUMOULIN, J. G., and BAGSHAWE, K. D., Pregnancy following choriocarcinoma. *J. Obstet. Gynec. Brit. Cwlth* 70, 1068—1072 (1963).

JACOBSON, W., Folic acid antagonists and cell division. *Pathologie-Biologie* 9, 481 (1961).

SAMPEY, J. R., 6-Mercaptopurine in combination chemotherapy of acute leukaemia. *Int. Rec.Med.* 174, 297—302 (1961).

SCHMORL, G., Über das Schicksal embolisch verschleppter Plazentarzellen. *Verh. dtsch. path. Ges.* 8, 39—46 (1904).

SUNG, H. C., WU, P. C., and HO, T. H., Treatment of choriocarcinoma and chorioadenoma destruens with 6-mercaptopurine and surgery. A clinical report of 93 cases. *Chin. med. J.* 82, 24—38 (1963).

WERKHEISER, W. C., The biochemical, cellular, and pharmacological action and effects of the folic acid antagonists. *Cancer Res.* 23, 1277—1285 (1963).

WILDE, C. E., ORR, H., and BAGSHAWE, K. D., Radioimmunoassay for chorionic gonadotrophin. *Nature (Lond.)* 205, 191—192 (1965).

WOODLIFF, H. J., The effect of antimetabolites on the respiration of leukaemic mouse cells. *Blood* 22, 199—208 (1963).

Remissions Induced in Patients with Trophoblastic Tumors by 6-Diazo-5-Oxo-L-Norleucine (DON)*

D. A. KARNOFSKY, R. B. GOLBEY, and M. C. LI

The Division of Clinical Chemotherapy, Sloan-Kettering Institute for Cancer Research, the Department of Medicine, Memorial and James Ewing Hospitals, and Cornell University Medical College, New York, New York

Trophoblastic tumors associated with pregnancy comprise a fascinating spectrum of diseases. Several aspects of these tumors relate directly to major problems in cancer research and therapy. These include, as examples, the transformations from normal cells to various levels of neoplasia in a single tissue; normal regression of disseminated benign trophoblastic tissues as contrasted with choriocarcinoma which is invasive and usually grows progressively; the spontaneous regression of metastatic trophoblastic tumors as a possible manifestation of host resistance, perhaps enhanced by an immunological incompatibility between the tumor, which is of fetal origin, and the maternal host; and finally the production of chorionic gonadotropic hormone by the tumor, which, also can serve as an index of tumor growth and regression.

When results from hysterectomy (BREWER et al., 1963) are constrasted to results with methotrexate (HERTZ et al., 1961; LI et al., 1956) and actinomycin D (Ross et al., 1962) it is apparent that progress has been made. It seems likely that with appropriate and aggressive chemotherapy about 2/3 of patients with metastatic trophoblastic tumors may be cured. Other drugs have been reported to produce remissions; these include the alkylating agents (KARNOFSKY et al., 1955), vinblastine HERTZ et al., 1960), and 6-mercaptopurine (SUNG et al., 1964). Susceptibility of trophoblastic tumors to chemotherapy does not seem to be related so much to the specific drug as to a peculiarly insecure position some of these tumors occupy in the host, which permits growth-inhibiting drugs to dislodge them successfully.

One of the reasons for the initial trial of the folic acid antagonist was the work of THIERSCH showing that aminopterin was selectively toxic to the rat fetus (1950) and to the human fetus (1952). It is thus postulated that aminopterin, or related antifolic derivatives, or other drugs toxic to the fetus in animals and man, might also be effective against trophoblastic tumors.

Table I lists drugs which have been used in trophoblastic tumors, and their selective toxicities to the rat embryo, adapted from Murphy's data (MURPHY, 1962). The LD50's for the maternal host as compared to the dose which inhibits

---

* The work reported in this article was supported in part by research grants CA-03215 and CA-05826 from the National Cancer Institute, Public Health Service, Department of Health, Education and Welfare.

fetal growth are shown. It is noted that, in some cases, there is a great difference between fetal and maternal toxicity, and DON appears to have the highest ratio.

DON, 6-diazo-5-oxo-L-norleucine, is an antibiotic and a glutamine analogue closely related to azaserine (3). Although this drug has a broad antitumor spectrum in experimental animals it has been largely ineffective against cancer in man (MAGILL et al., 1957; MYERS and MAGILL, 1956).

The tolerated dosage is well-established, and it is equally active when administered by mouth or intramuscularly. Its chief toxic manifestations are the appearance of redness of the tongue and mucous membranes, diarrhea, nausea and vomiting, and occasionally mild hematologic depression. DON is thus a relatively safe drug, and bone marrow depression is not one of its major actions.

BUCHANAN and his colleagues (1959) have shown that DON interferes with the transfer of amino groups from glutamine, in the synthetic steps from [1] formylglycineamide ribotide to formylglycineamidine ribotide, from [2] phosphoribosylpyrophosphate to phosphoribosylamine, as well as in other amination reactions. DON, thus, appears to act principally by interfering with purine biosynthesis, but other mechanisms may be involved to explain the remarkable susceptibility of embryonic tissue.

We have treated 11 patients with trophoblastic tumors with DON over the past 7 years. Following our first two responses to DON, HERTZ and his group in 1958 reported that DON failed to produce any effect in 4 patients with methotrexate-resistant choriocarcinoma (HERTZ et al., 1958). Our data suggest that DON has a definite therapeutic effect on previously untreated trophoblastic tumors; treatment for 3 to 6 weeks is necessary to produce a satisfactory re-

sponse, but it should be continued for a considerably longer period.

Dosage

DON is initially given orally at a dose of 0.5 mg/kg daily (25—40 mg) in three divided doses. Patients may complain of a little gastrointestinal irritation, but the most significant symptom is a

Table I. *Effects of drugs, used in the treatment of trophoblastic tumors, on the rat fetus*

	Estimated fetal: maternal toxicity ratio	Teratogenic activity
Nitrogen mustard	1 : 4	+
Methotrexate	1 : 100	±
DON	1 : 800	±
6-MP	1 : 6	+
Vinblastine	1 : 4	±
Actinomycin D	1 : 1.5	±

sore, bright red tongue which occurs in 7 to 10 days. The dose is then interrupted for a day or two, and the red tongue promptly subsides. Treatment is then continued at a lower dose (15—20 mg/day) and a maintenance dose is established. The patient learns to increase or decrease the dosage depending on how her tongue feels. After the chorionic gonadotropin levels have fallen to a normal level and all signs of the disease have disappeared, DON has been continued for an additional 4 to 6 months, and then stopped. One of the problems after stopping the treatment has been persistent scarring at the site of pulmonary metastases. If the urinary titer is normal, and the pulmonary lesions are not progressing, treatment has been stopped six months after the pulmonary lesion has become stabilized.

Results

Table II lists the seven patients who have responded favorably to DON.

Table II. *Favorable responses to DON in patients without prior chemotherapy*

Patient/ Age	Diagnosis	Prior to DON therapy				After DON	
		Duration (Months)	Surgery	PS[1]	Titer[2] x 10³ I. U.	Response	Duration (Years)
Local disease							
BD/ 49	Invasive mole	5	H[3]	90	500	C[4]	7 $^{3}/_{12}$
UH/ 31	Invasive mole	6	H	90	40	C	2 $^{4}/_{12}$
HC/ 19	Hydatid mole	19	L[5]	100	.3	C	1
Pulmonary metastases							
CV/ 25	Trophoblastic neoplasia	5	H	90	10	C	7
EC/ 25	Invasive and metastatic mole	2	H	90	3	C	3 $^{3}/_{12}$
CM/ 52	Choriocarcinoma	4	H	80	50	C	1 $^{6}/_{12}$
MG/ 21	Metastatic mole	3	—	70	50	C	$^{10}/_{12}$

[1] PS: performance status.
[2] Titer $\times$ 10³ I. U.: urinary chorionic gonadotropin titre — international units.
[3] H: hysterectomy.
[4] C: complete.
[5] L: laparotomy.

Three apparently had persistent local disease (two following hysterectomy) and the diagnosis was based mainly on a persistently elevated urinary gonadotropin titer. The first patient (BD) also had a mass, palpable by pelvic examination, in the pelvic floor. These patients, who had received no previous chemotherapy, showed a complete response.

Four patients had x-ray evidence of pulmonary metastases and an elevated hormone titer which persisted, in three cases, following hysterectomy. In all of these cases, the urinary titer returned to normal in 4 to 6 weeks of treatment (Fig. 1). Treatment, however, was continued for at least six months after the titer became normal and there has been no evidence of recurrent disease. In two cases (CM and MG), there are faint persistent scars which are observed on x-ray examination of the lungs.

Four patients failed to respond satisfactorily to DON therapy (Table III); two patients were initially treated with DON (MD and SZ) (Fig. 2). MD, a 26 year old obese female, had a curettage in January, 1958. Two months later, because of persistent vaginal bleeding, a laparotomy revealed a widely infiltrating choriocarcinoma involving the uterus, rectum and bladder. A non-functioning right kidney on intravenous pyelography, and pulmonary metastases were present. There was also definite biochemical evidence of liver involvement. The patient received DON from March 17 to May 4, 1958 without improvement. A course of an alkylating agent, epoxypiperazine, produced leukopenia and thrombocytopenia and the patient died of overwhelming sepsis and a cerebral hemorrhage. At autopsy, the disease was diagnosed as chorioadenoma destruens.

SZ, a 22 year old female, had an incomplete abortion in May, 1962 with persistent evidence of trophoblastic activity. In September, 1963, the patient had a curettage and proliferative endometrium was found. In May, 1964, she de-

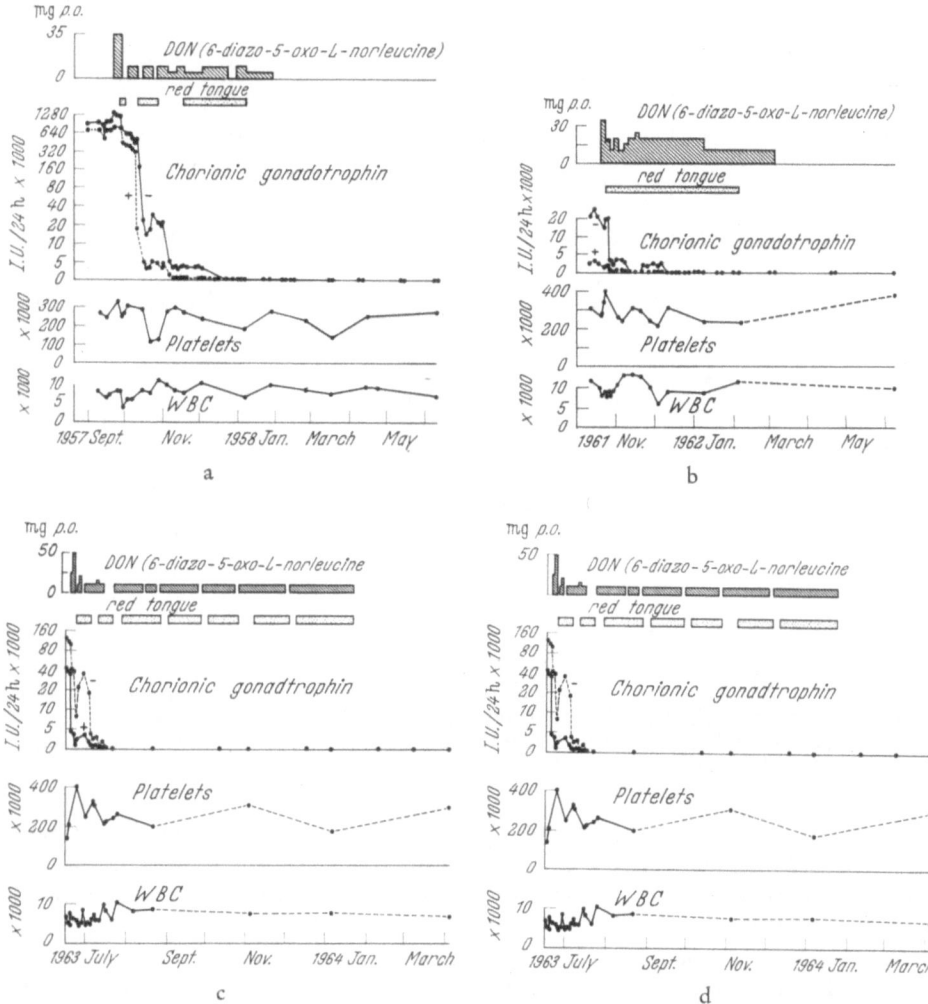

Fig. 1a—d. a B. D. 49 year old female, diagnosis chorioadenoma destruens. Prior to chemotherapy the patient had a D and C (4/57), hysterectomy and salpingo-oophorectomy (6/21/57). b E. C. 25 year old female, diagnosis chorioadenoma destruens. Prior to chemotherapy the patient had a D and C (8/12, 8/26/61), hysterectomy and lt. salpingo-oophorectomy (8/30/61). c C. M. 52 year old female, diagnosis choriocarcinoma. Prior to chemotherapy the patient had a D and C (4/63) and hysterectomy (5/13/63). d M. G. 21 year old female, diagnosis trophoblastic tumor of uterus. Prior to chemotherapy the patient had a D and C (1/6/64, 3/8/64)

veloped bilateral pulmonary metastases, and liver involvement. A hysterectomy, at this time, showed choriocarcinoma (Fig. 2). The patient received DON for one week at high doses, but showed no change in her gonadotropin titer and her pulmonary symptoms progressed so that she became critically ill with severe dyspnea. She then received actinomycin D, Thio TEPA, and methotrexate with a prompt response. After improvement occurred, she was maintained on DON, but relapsed with an increase in pulmonary metastases and gonadotropin titer.

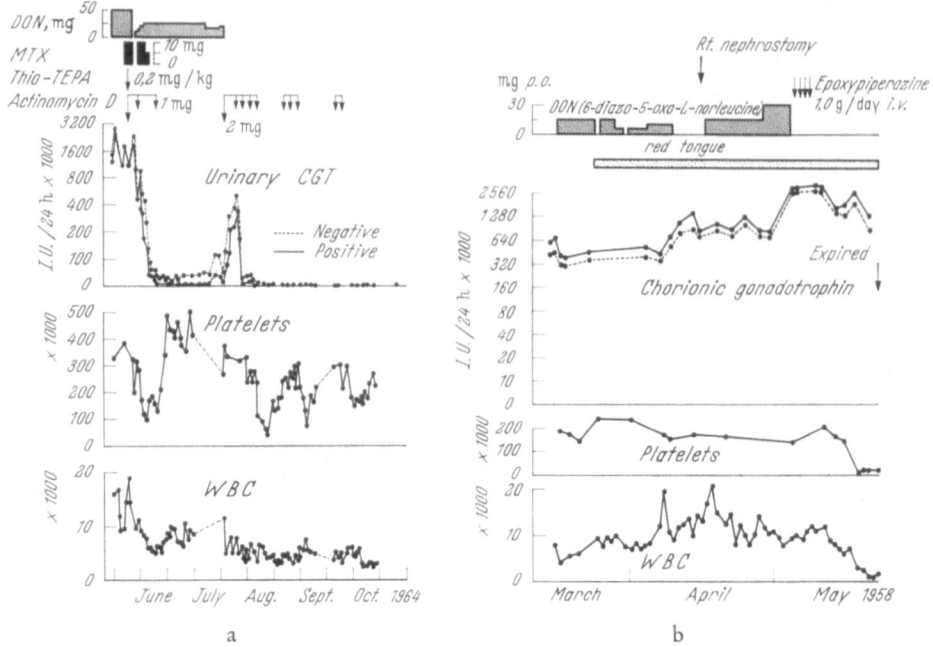

Fig. 2a and b. a S. Z. 22 year old female, diagnosis choriocarcinoma. Prior to chemotherapy the patient had a D and C (5/62, 9/63), laparotomy (9/63), panhysterectomy (5/64). b M. D. 26 year old female, diagnosis chorioadenoma destruens. Prior to chemotherapy the patient had a D and C (1/16/58), laparotomy (2/2/58), cystotomy (2/26/58), D and C (3/5/58)

Actinomycin D caused prompt improvement, and she is now receiving intermittent courses of actinomycin D with complete control of the disease. This patient failed to respond to DON.

In addition, two patients resistant to methotrexate have died following DON. One patient, MB, had a hydatid mole for about 16 months with repeated recurrences. After choriocarcinoma with generalized metastases developed, she received methotrexate, vinblastine, 6-mercaptopurine and actinomycin D with only transient improvement. The patient was treated with DON for two weeks without improvement and she died of myocardial failure secondary to the pulmonary metastases. The second patient, SK, showed only transient improvement in her urinary titer on methotrexate, and the pulmonary metastases progressed. On

DON, which the patient did not take regularly, there was only transient and minimal benefit. She refused a course of actinomycin D and returned to her native country where she died without further therapy. She is regarded as a DON failure.

Discussion

DON appeared to be effective against hydatid mole and chorioadenoma destruens in 7 cases; 4 patients in the group with pulmonary metastases, as demonstrated by x-ray examination of the chest, showed complete regression. These patients were in good general condition with slowly progressive disease, and were previously untreated, except for hysterectomy in 5/7 cases. A complete response required 3 to 6 weeks of treatment, and the patients were then readily maintained

Table III. *Failures on DON therapy*

Patient/ Age	Diagnosis	Prior to DON therapy					After DON
		Duration (Months)	Chemo- therapy	Surgery	PS[1]	Titer[3] $\times 10^3$ I. U.	Response
Pulmonary metastases and local							
SK/ 20	Chorio- carcinoma	30	MTX[4]	—	80	300	Transient response died 6 months
MD/ 26	Chorio- carcinoma	1	0	L[5]	50	300	No response died 2 months
MB/ 25	Mole Chorio- carcinoma	26 10	MTX VLB[6] Act.D[7] 6—MP[8]	H[2]	60	1420	No response died 2 weeks
SZ/ 22	Chorio- carcinoma	15	0	H	40	1600	DON failure; response to actinomycin D

[1] PS: performance status.
[2] H: hysterectomy.
[3] Titer $\times 10^3$ I. U.: urinary chorionic gonadotropin titre — international units.
[4] MTX: methotrexate.
[5] L: laparotomy.
[6] VLB: vinblastine.
[7] Act. D: actinomycin D.
[8] 6-MP: 6-mercaptopurine.

on prolonged DON therapy. Spontaneous regressions do occur and the favorable responses in an individual case cannot be attributed necessarily to DON (17). The consistent results obtained, however suggest that DON is effective against these tumors.

DON, however, was ineffective in the two patients resistant to methotrexate, and this would presumably be the case in patients refractory to other drugs active against trophoblastic tumors. HERTZ, et al., (1958) made a similar observation. Furthermore, DON, as the initial form of treatment, was not effective against highly malignant and widely disseminated trophoblastic tumors in either of two patients. Our data indicate that these patients should be treated with more active drugs, such as metho-

trexate and actinomycin D (Ross et al., 1962).

In Figure 3 the role of the several drugs effective in trophoblastic tumors has been summarized for purposes of discussion. The course of the disease is plotted against time and while a hydatid mole may progress from a noninvasive to an invasive form, and then to a choriocarcinoma, these transitions are infrequently observed. The course in the individual patient may be quite different. In Figure 3, the A line refers to a hydatid mole which regresses spontaneously; B to the mole which is initially invasive; C to the trophoblastic tumor which appears from the onset as choriocarcinoma and D to the mole which progresses steadily to high levels of neoplasia. A drug active against choriocarcinoma would presumably be effective in the less malignant manifestations of the disease. At the upper portion of Figure 3, actinomycin D is noted as the drug of first choice. Its effectiveness has been demonstrated in rapidly progressive choriocarcinoma. It appears to be safer in general use than the high daily dose schedule of methotrexate and impaired renal function does not increase the toxicity of actinomycin D, as in the case of methotrexate. Methotrexate may be equally effective in many

iocarcinoma. DON, as a relatively safe agent, may be indicated in patients with hydatid mole to prevent the evolution of the more malignant forms of trophoblastic tumors. DON, if effective, should reduce an elevated chorionic gonadotropin titer to normal levels within 3 to 6 weeks; an elevated titer after 2 months on DON would suggest serious trophoblastic disease. If DON proved to be equally as effective as methotrexate, it would be a much safer agent for general

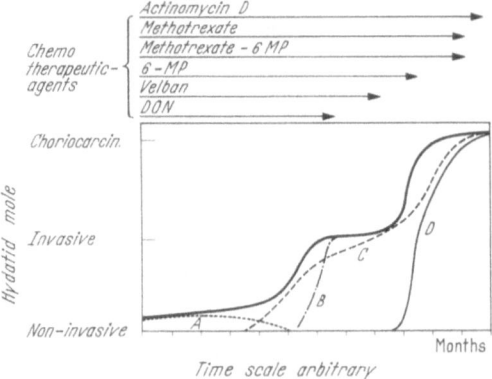

Fig. 3. Schedule of treatment for various stages of trophoblastic neoplasia

cases, and the methotrexate-6 mercaptopurine combination is highly effective, and may produce less danger of systemic toxicity since smaller doses of methotrexate are used. Mercaptopurine and vinblastine may possibly be less active generally, but they have been effective in choriocarcinoma. DON has only been useful up to the invasive mole level in our experience.

In rapidly growing choriocarcinoma the most effective drug should be used, to give the greatest possibility of permanent control, while the development of resistance and of subsequent relapse is reduced to a minimum. DON, or one of its analogues, may prove to be useful in the invasive and non-invasive moles.

Hydatid moles have a substantial risk of becoming invasive or developing chor-

use in non-metastatic trophoblastic neoplasia with the aim of preserving reproductive function.

The relationship between the mechanism of action of anti-cancer drugs, the histology and biological behavior of trophoblastic tumors and their response to treatment may lead to significant observations on the reasons for the unique curabiliy of these tumors by chemotherapy. Certain anti-cancer drugs have been given during normal pregnancy without serious injury to the placenta as judged by fetal survival with normal development (KARNOFSKY, 1965). Normal trophoblastic cells, metastatic to the lungs, are apparently readily destroyed by a systemic mechanism whereas trophoblastic tumor cells are not. Is complete regression of trophoblastic tumor cells following chemotherapy due (a) to direct cytotoxic effects on the tumor cells, (b) to damage to the cellular mechanism whereby the trophoblast protects itself from a hostile environment, or (c) to an immunological mechanism acting on the cells surviving the chemotherapy?

At present, DON is not available in quantity, and it is more difficult to synthesize than its closely related analogue, O-diazoacetyl-L-serine (azaserine) (ELLISON et al., 1954). Azaserine is about 1/50 as active as DON by weight, and the usual daily dose is in the range of 10 to 15 mg/kg (500—1000 mg/day). The toxic effects of DON and azaserine in man have been compared by MAGILL, et al. At equivalent pharmacological doses, they are quite similar in their effects on the oral mucosa. Azaserine causes a higher incidence of gastrointestinal symptoms, and 15 per cent of the patients developed disturbances in liver function. It would be desirable to study azaserine in trophoblastic tumors, since it may be equal or perhaps even more effective than DON, and adequate supplies of azaserine are easier to manufacture.

Conclusions

DON (6-diazo-5-oxo-L-norleucine) is an antimetabolite, which acts by inhibiting the functions of glutamine in purine biosynthesis. It has a high safety margin in man, and its major toxicity is reddening of the tongue and oral mucosa.

DON produced therapeutic effects on 7 of 11 patients with trophoblastic tumors with elevated urinary chorionic gonadotropin levels; 4 of the patients who responded had x-ray evidence of pulmonary metastases. Four patients did not respond; 2 were resistant to methotrexate, and 2 had rapidly progressive and widely metastatic disease.

The role of DON, in relation to the other anti-cancer drugs effective against choriocarcinoma, is not yet defined. It is not indicated in aggressive and widely disseminated choriocarcinoma; actinomycin D and methotrexate act more rapidly and are therapeutically more effective. DON may prove to be safe and effective against invasive and non-invasive moles and it may be that it could be used early to prevent the threat of a more malignant form of trophoblastic tumor.

References

BREWER, J. I., SMITH, R. T., and PRATT, G. B., Choriocarcinoma. Absolute 5 year survival rates of 122 patients treated by hysterectomy. *Amer. J. Obstet. Gynec.* **85**, 841—843 (1963).

BUCHANAN, J. M., HARTMAN, S. C., HERRMANN, R. L., and DAY, R. A.; Reactions involving the carbon-nitrogen bond: heterocyclic compounds. *J. cell. comp. Physiol.* **54**, 139—160 (1959).

CLARKE, D. A., REILLY, H. C., and STOCK, C. C., Comparative study of 6-diazo-5-oxo-L-norleucine and O-diazoacetyl-L-serine on sarcoma 180. *Proc. Amer. Ass. Cancer Res.* **2**, 100 (1956).

ELLISON R. R., KARNOFSKY, D. A., STERNBERG, S. S., MURPHY, M. L., and BURCHENAL, J. H., Clinical trials of O-diazoacetyl-L-serine (azaserine) in neoplastic disease. *Cancer* (Philad.) **1**, 801—814 (1954).

HERTZ, R., Personal communication.

— BERGENSTAL, D. M., LIPSETT, M. B., PRICE, E. G., and HILBISH, T. F., Chemotherapy of choriocarcinoma and related trophoblastic tumors in women. *J. Amer. med. Ass.* **168**, 845—854 (1958).

— LEWIS, J., Jr., and LIPSETT, M. B., Five years' experience with the chemotherapy of metastatic choriocarcinoma and related trophoblastic tumors in women. *Amer. J. Obstet. Gynec.* **82**, 631—640 (1961).

—, LIPSETT, M. B., and MOY, R. H., Effect of vincaleukoblastine on metastatic choriocarcinoma and related trophoblastic tumors in women. *Cancer Res.* **20**, 1050—1053 (1960).

KARNOFSKY, D. A., Drugs as teratogens in animals and man. *Ann. Rev. Pharmacol.* **5**, 447—472 (1965).

Karnofsky, D. A., Myers, W. P. L., and Phillips, R., Treatment of the inoperable pulmonary cancer primary and metastatic. *Amer. J. Surg.* **89**, 526—537 (1955).

Li, M. C., Hertz, R., and Spencer, D. B., Effect of methotrexate therapy upon choriocarcinoma and chorioadenoma. *Proc. Soc. exp. Biol. (N. Y.)* **93**, 361—366 (1956).

Magill, G. B., Myers, W. P. L., Reilly, H. C., Putnam, R. C., Magill, J. W., Sykes, M. P., Escher, G. C., Karnofsky, D. A., and Burchenal, J. H., Pharmacological and initial therapeutic observations on 6-diazo-5-oxo-L-norleucine (DON) in human neoplastic disease. *Cancer (Philad.)* **10**, 1138—1150 (1957).

Murphy, M. L., Teratogenic effects in rats of growth inhibiting chemicals, including studies on thalidomide. *Clin. Proc. Child. Hosp. (Wash.)* **18**, 307—322 (1962).

Myers, W. P. L., and Magill, G. B., Alterations in calcium metabolism in cancer patients treated with 6-diazo-5-oxo-L-norleucine. *Proc. Soc. exp. Biol. (N. Y.)* **93**, 314—318 (1956).

Ross, G. T., Stalbach, L. L., and Hertz, R., Actinomycin D in the treatment of methotrexate-resistant trophoblastic disease in women. *Cancer Res.* **22**, 1015—1017 (1962).

Sung, H-c., Wu, P-c, and Ho, T-h., Treatment of choriocarcinoma and chorioadenoma destruens with 6-mercaptopurine and sugery. *Acta Un. int. Cancr.* **20**, 493—502 (1964).

Thiele, R. A., and de Alvarez. R. R., Metastasizing benign trophoblastic tumors. *Amer. J. Obstet. Gynec.* **84**, 1395—1406 (1962).

Thiersch, J. B., Therapeutic abortions with a folic acid antagonist 4-amino-pteroylglutamic acid (4-amino P. G. A.) administered by the oral route. *Amer. J. Obstet. Gynec.* **63**, 1298—1304 (1952).

—, and Phillips, F. S., Effect of 4-aminopteroylglutamic acid (aminopterin) in early pregnancy. *Proc. Soc. exp. Biol. (N. Y.)* **74**, 204—208 (1950).

Trophoblast and its tumors. *Ann. N. Y. Acad. Sci.* **80**, 1—284 (1959).

Fundamental Problems of Chemotherapy of Choriocarcinoma

Misao Natsume

Department of Obstretics and Gynecology
University of Gifu School of Medicine, Gifu, Japan

Based on experience with more than 10 patients with choriocarcinoma treated with amethopterin and vinblastine the following presumptive conclusions are reached. Chorionic tumors may present explosive pulmonary growth 10 days after hysterectomy. This may represent accelerated growth in previously dormant lesions, or new embolic metastases. Chemotherapy should be used as early as possible in the course of the disease. It should be used prior to surgical therapy to counteract tumor development and dissemination which might be accelerated by the surgery. Chemotherapy, by promoting regression, may make surgery easier, or unnecessary. Immune mechanisms may be involved in this regression, and should, if possible, be potentiated. Whenever appropriate, the gross tumor should be extirpated to improve host tumor relationship. Chorionic tumors should be regarded as a generalizing disease, always exfoliating tumor cells into the circulation. Thus chemotherapy should be used before and after surgery. The author's views were supported with case presentations.

Clinical Effects of Vinblastine in Chorionic Tumors

Toshio Hasegawa, M. D., Genichi Ogawa, M. D., Takashi Kobayashi, M. D.,
Misao Natsume, M. D., Yoshio Ashidaka, M. D., Kohachiro Koga, M. D.,
and Genichi Nozue, M. D.

*Chorionic Tumor Committee, the Japanese
Obstetrical and Gynecological Society, Japan*

In a cooperative study by selected members of the Chorionic Tumor Committee, the Japanese Obstetrical and Gynecological Society, Japan, 40 patients were treated with Vinblastine Sulfate. Twelve of these had chorionepithelioma [choriocarcinoma — Ed.] 16 had destructive mole [invasive hydatidiform mole — Ed.] and 12 had hydatidiform mole. Final diagnosis was based on histologic findings which had been agreed upon at a special session of the Chorionic Tumor Committee.

Most of the patients were initially given 0.1—0.15 mg of vinblastine per kg body weight in the tubing of a rapidly running infusion at one week intervals. Subsequently, doses were increased to 0.2 mg/kg twice a week if no untoward effect was observed. The interval between injections varied somehat from patient to patient, to minimize unfavorable side effects. Additional therapy consisted of appropriate surgery and other anticancer drugs e. g. amethopterin, nitromin, cyclophosphamide, and mitomycin.

On vinblastine, leukopenia occurred in 20 and thrombocytopenia in 4 out of 37 patients. No gastrointestinal toxicity and no epilation was noted. The therapeutic results were evaluated by changes in chorionic gonadotropin titers (expressed by rabbit units in Friedman test), physical findings and symptoms. Seven out of 12 patients with chorionepithelioma and 14 out of 28 patients with noninvasive and invasive mole were thought to have derived some measure of benefit from treatment with vinblastine. The potential value of vinblastine in prophylaxis of development of chorionepithelioma could not be determined because of the brief followup period in patients with hydatidiform mole.

The Clinical Evaluation of Various Anticancer Agents on Chorionic Tumors

Professor TAKASHI KOBAYASHI, M. D.

The Department of Obstetrics and Gynecology
Tokyo University School of Medicine

From 1953 to 1963 76 cases of chorionic tumors were treated. All patients with invasive mole or chorioepithelioma except one were treated by hysterectomy; 39 of these patients consisting of 11 cases with invasive mole (chorioadenoma destruens) and 28 cases with choriocarcinoma, received chemotherapy postoperatively. Nitrogen mustard N-oxide in a dose of 1 mg/kg per day for 10—20 days was used in 21 patients and it was judged to be effective in 13, but only one of ten patients with metastatic choriocarcinoma showed a good response. Cyclophosphamide in a dose of 2 mg/kg per day for 20—40 days was administered to 15 patients, and 12 of them responded effectively; 2 of 7 patients with metastatic choriocarcinoma had a good response. Amethopterin 10—20 mg per day for 5—10 days was given to 7 patients, and 6 of them had a good response responses; 1 of 2 patients with metastatic choriocarcinoma had a good effect. Other drugs also used were Mitomycin, Toyomycin, and TESPA.

The three year survival rate was studied for 61 patients thus treated during the first seven years. In this period of time no Amethopterin was used in any of these patients. The overall survival rate in 22 patients with invasive mole (chorioadenoma destruens) was 86.4 per cent, 90 per cent in 10 patients who received chemotherapy and 83.3 per cent in those who did not. The overall survival rate in 39 choriocarcinoma patients was 46 per cent, 50 per cent in patients receiving and 42.8 per cent in patients not receiving chemotherapy. Of two patients with metastatic invasive mole, one patient received chemotherapy and died, and the other survived without chemotherapy. Of 12 patients with metastatic choriocarcinoma who received chemotherapy 3 survived (25 per cent). Of 13 not receiving chemotherapy, 2 survived (15 per cent).

These data may indicate that the tumor type and the spread of the disease, rather than chemotherapy adjuvant to surgery were the determining factors in the outcome of the disease. As far as Amethopterin is concerned, a conclusion will be obtained in further studies.

Chemotherapeutic and Immunological Considerations on the Response of Choriocarcinomas*

Min C. Li, M. D.

Nassau Hospital, Mineola, N. Y.

Choriocarcinoma can originate either from the products of conception, or from the germinal cells of the gonads of either sex. Rarely, it may arise from embryonal rest cells in extra-gonadal sites such as the

Table: I. *Difference in folic acid requirements for growth of transplanted testicular and uterine choriocarcinoma in hamsters.*

	Take	%
A. *Folic acid deficient diet + vegetables + fruits*		
Uterine choriocarcinoma (W. O.)	26/56	46
Testis choriocarcinoma (Pitt 89)	47/78	60
B. *Folic acid deficient diet*		
Uterine choriocarcinoma (W. O.)	6/44	14
Testis choriocarcinoma (Pitt 89)	56/86	65
C. *Folic acid deficient diet + folic acid*		
Uterine choriocarcinoma (W. O.)	6/10	60

mediastinum, pineal body, lung, stomach, urinary bladder, and tissues in the retroperitoneal area. Although choriocarcinoma of different origins are similar in their histological appearance, in the production of chorionic gonadotropin and in their clinical behaviour and rapid dissemination, they respond differently to chemotherapeutic agents and they differ in their host-tumor relationships. The present report deals with the findings of investigations on these two topics.

Uterine choriocarcinoma is sensitive to methotrexate, actinomycin D, 6-mercaptopurine, 6-diazo-5-oxo-L-norleucine, and some of the alkylating agents. Choriocarcinomas of gonadal or extra-gonadal origin, have, on the contrary, not responded regularly and satisfactorily to these drugs when given singly in our experience (Li *et al.* 1958, 1960). At first the question of difference of hormonal influence was entertained as being a responsible factor for the lack of effect of these drugs on non-gestational tumors. This was later clearly ruled out as a possibility by experiments exemplified in the following study. Figure 1 represents the determinations of urinary chorionic gonadotropin during the course of study on a man who had multiple choriocarcinoma metastases in both lungs shortly after a unilateral orchiectomy to remove the primary tumor. Before he was treated with Methotrexate the remaining testis was removed to eliminate a major source of androgen secretion. He was then given two five-day courses of metho-

* This study was supported in part by grants from the American Cancer Society.

trexate which induced no effect on chorionic gonadotropin excretion. After this, he was placed on a massive dose of estrogen daily, and methotrexate was repeated but was without effect. Similar studies were made on three other patients. The output of urinary chorionic gonado-

periments. In these experiments, both uterine choriocarcinoma (WO strain)[1] and testicular choriocarcinoma (Pitt 89)[2], were transplanted respectively to the cheek pouches of cortisonized hamsters which had been maintained on a folic deficient diet for at least three weeks

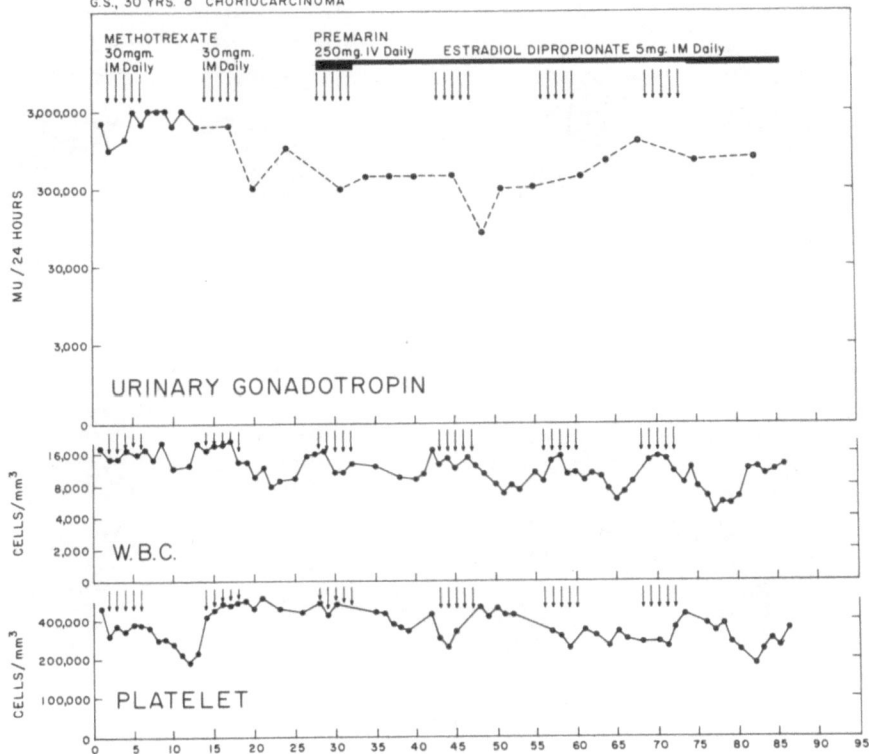

Fig. 1. Effect of orchiectomy and estrogen with or without methotrexate therapy on testis choriocarcinoma

tropin and metastatic lesions were not influenced by the therapy which would have been effective against gestational choriocarcinoma in most cases.

The difference in growth requirement for folic acid between uterine and testicular choriocarcinoma was our second consideration. This was not clarified until we were able to transplant and maintain growth of these two human tumors in the cheek pouches of cortisonized hamsters. Table I summarizes thes results of our ex-

prior to experimentation. As indicated in Table I, the percentage of takes of uterine choriocarcinoma was substantially higher when folate was in the diet (A &C) than when it was omitted. Testicular choriocarcinoma transplantability was independent of diet, however (A & B) suggesting that folic acid is not as essential

---

[1] Courtesy of Dr. R. HERTZ of the National Cancer Institute.

[2] Courtesy of Dr. BARRY Pierce of the University of Michigan Medical School.

for growth of testicular choriocarcinoma as it is for uterine choriocarcinoma.

The failure of reponse of testicular choriocarcinoma to the drugs mentioned previously, has led us to explore the effect of combinations of drugs. After many clinical trials, a feasible triple drug re-

(0.5 mg. each dose) are given intravenously with a five-day resting period between each course. Although the majority of patients tolerated the regimen well, not infrequently drug toxicity developed prior to the end of the planned regimen, necessitating termination of drug therapy.

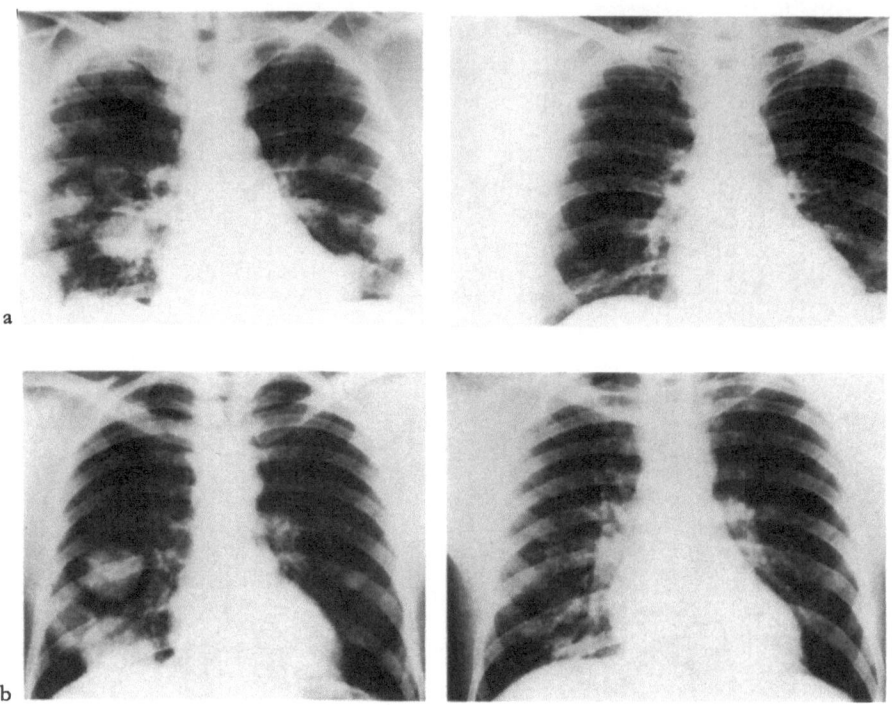

Fig. 2

Fig. 2 a (upper two). Roentgenograph evidences of tumor regression fellowing triple drug therapy. Patient: L. M. C.
Fig. 2 b (lower two). Roentgenograph evidence of tumor regression following triple drug therapy. Patient: D. C.

gimen was devised (Li et al., 1960). This regimen is aimed at rendering maximum deleterious effect on embryonal tissues by different mechanisms through the combination of three classes of teratogenic agents, namely, chlorambucil, Methotrexate, and Actinomycin D. The drug regimen consists of Chlorambucil, 10 mgm., and Methotrexate, 5 mgm., given daily by mouth for 25 days. In addition, three five-day courses of Actinomycin D

Drug toxicity, such as hematological depression, oral ulceration, diarrhea and loss of hair, are generally short-lasting and reversible. Extreme caution must be exercised in patients who show pre-existing impairment of functions of the bone marrow, liver or kidneys, however, for under such conditions toxicity is likely to be greatly augmented.

Figure 2a shows the roentgenographic evidence of response to therapy of a man having numerous metastases from choriocarcinoma and teratocarcinoma of the testis to both lungs. The response is dramatic but transient, lasting only six months. Accompanying this, his urinary chorionic gonadotropin titre declined from 300,000 I. U. per day to negative values, following therapy. Figure 2b shows the remarkable response of another man with metastatic testicular choriocarcinoma in both lungs. His urinary chorionic gonadotropin titre receded from 650,000 I. U. to negative values. This patient has been completely free of evidence of disease for six years.

Dr. A. R. MACKENZIE (1964) at Memorial Hospital in New York has recently reviewed 72 patients with various types of metastatic testicular cancer, including teratocarcinoma and embryonal carcinoma and seminoma. This triple drug regimen or its modification induced tumor regression or diminution of urinary chorionic gonadotropin titre in 50 % of these 72 patients, although the majority of effects were transient in nature. Of the responders, only seven showed complete disappearance of all metastatic tumors and return of high chorionic gonadotropin titre, when present, to negative values. In spite of maintenance therapy, rarely can complete tumor regression be sustained longer than two years. Three of these seven have gone five to six years without evidence of disease.

Our experience with mithramycin in the treatment of metastatic testicular carcinoma is rather limited. Thus far we have not seen favorable results in five patients. However, in a recent review of literature on the effect of mithramycin in the treatment of metastatic testicular cancer, BROWN and KENNEDY (1965) stated that 22 out of 46 patients showed objective regression. Some of these responders had choriocarcinoma.

The rarity of attaining complete tumor regression with testicular choriocarcinoma in contrast to uterine choriocarcinoma has stimulated us to study the differences in immunological aspects of the two diseases. Uterine trophoblastic tumor is the product of the conceptus, genetically consisting of maternal as well as paternal components. The host-tumor relationship is thus similar to homologous transplants and is theoretically subject to rejection. This assumption is supported by the spontaneous regression of this tumor occasionally noted. Admittedly, the antigenicity of trophoblastic tissue may be a doubtful one in the same species and the mother can develop tolerance to the graft. On the other hand, the host-tumor relationship of metastatic testicular choriocarcinoma is that of an autograft and, therefore, no immunological rejection of the tumor is expected.

If the host-tumor relationship with uterine choriocarcinoma is truly that of a homologous graft, one would expect accelerated rejection when skin of the husband or children is grafted to the patient. In a patient with active metastatic uterine choriocarcinoma, a graft from her husband, an autograft, a graft from an unrelated person, and a graft from the patient's daughter were placed. Five weeks after transplantation the autograft had taken well; grafts from her husband, daughter and the unrelated person showed no rejection at this time. We have had similar grafts on another woman with active metastatic uterine choriocarcinoma showing similar results. Although these data at first were a big surprise to us, nevertheless, they confirm the observations recently reported in the literature by ROBINSON et al., 1963 and by MATHE et al., 1964. The findings of a delayed homograft rejection by patients with uterine choriocarcinoma are compatible with the general phenomenon of tolerance of skin homografts in cancer subjects observed by GRACE (1958). No specific tolerance to the husband's tissues need be postulated. The possibility of drug-induced tolerance has been avoided because the patients were not receiving therapy during the experimented period. To further clarify this point, we have made skin grafts of husband and an unrelated person to two other women who mechanisms of homograft rejection of the host with trophoblastic tumor suppressed? Why is the inhibition reversible when trophoblastic tumors are eliminated? It is possible that trophoblastic cells secrete some unknown substance that would suppress the normal homograft rejection mechanism, and does the trophoblastic

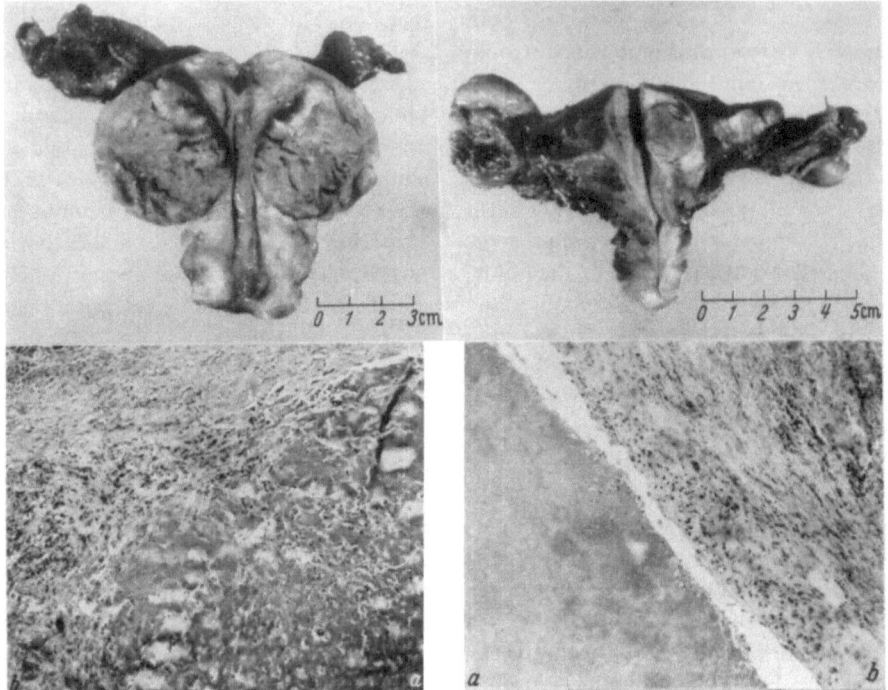

Fig. 3. The macroscopic and microscopie appearance of treated uterine choriocarcinoma. *a* tumor tissue; *b* myometrium

had had metastatic choriocarcinoma and have had complete remission of disease for four and five years after therapy. Complete rejection of the homografts occurred at the end of the third week. This is in complete agreement with the usual findings in homograft rejection by normal individuals.

Although these data can be interpreted as consistent with the findings in people who are and are not seriously ill with cancer, one can ask if specific features apply to trophoblastic tumors. Are the cell itself repel the infiltration of inflammatory cells? If there is such a substance, it must be species specific, for heterograft rejection of human gestational choriocarcinoma in non-cortisonized hamster cheeck pouch three weeks after implantation is characterized by a heavy infiltrate of inflammatory cells.

Careful microscopic examination of tumor tissue removed from patients during or after chemotherapy has been made seeking evidence of tissue reaction that may indicate the presence of an immunological interaction. Figure 3 (left) shows the macroscopic and microscopic appearances of a choriocarcinoma in the uterus which was removed from a patient shortly after completion of Methotrexate therapy. Her pulmonary metastases had regressed and her urinary chorionic gonadotropin titre had returned to negative values. The tumor shows diffuse necrotic, disintegrated cellular materials adjacent to the myometrium. Microscopically, one sees no evidence of monocyte, lymphocyte or plasma cell infiltration. Figure 3 (right)

effective against uterine choriocarcinoma are also immuno-suppressive. BREWER and PARK have each described untreated trophoblastic tumors showing absence of infiltration of inflammatory cells. HSU has a single case of inflammatory reaction surrounding tumor tissue in the brain.

Since skin homograft rejection does occur in women with trophoblastic tumor, although in a delayed manner, and complete spontaneous disappearance of trophoblastic tumors has been repeatedly demonstrated, one must be reconciled to

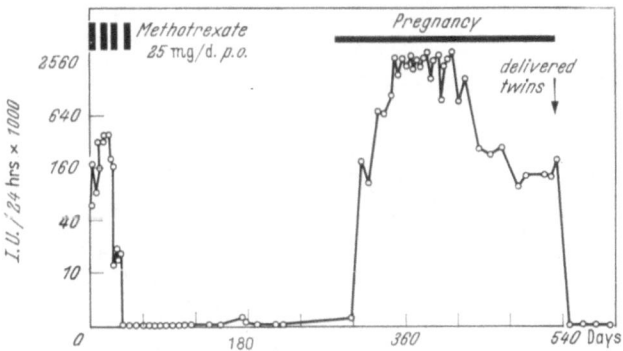

Fig. 4. Normal pregnancy following a treated uterine choriocarcinoma having complete tumor regression

shows the macroscopic and microscopic appearances of a choriocarcinoma in the uterus removed from a woman who had completed Methotrexate therapy three months previously. All measurable metastatic lesions in this patient had totally regressed and there was no detectable chorionic gonadotropin in the urine. Here again, one sees only homogenous eosinophilic materials. The junction between the tumor and myometrium was sharply demarcated. Microscopically, there was no evidence of lymphocyte, plasma cell or fibroblastic infiltration. It is also possible, however, that these cellular elements, commonly seen in tissues of autoimmune diseases and graft rejection, can be eliminated by the drugs used for therapy. It has been known that agents which are

the possibility that our body may have another immune mechanism to account for these phenomena. We all know that drug only exerts its effect by way of cytoxicity. The elimination of dead tumor cells remains in the realm of a process of self-defense.

An argument in strong support of the lack of antigenicity of trophoblastic cells perhaps can be found in those women who have had complete remission of widespread trophoblastic disease and have become pregnant later. Figure 4 shows the gonadotropin response of a young woman who had a choriocarcinoma in the uterus with metastasis to the vagina. Nine months after she had been in total remission of disease, she was pregnant. She had an uncomplicated gestation period and delivered normal twins at the end. A year later she was pregnant again, delivering another normal baby. These findings are contrary to those observed in erythroblastosis fetalis and suggest that choriocarcinomatous tissue may be entirely non-antigenic, or the anti-choriocarcinoma element in this woman may not be specific enough to cause damage to fetal tissues.

Since we have failed to come to a definite conclusion from experimental data by way of tissue reaction, whether

Despite the lack of evidence of a transplantation immunity in women with trophoblastic disease, we believe the reason for the sustained tumor regression following therapy is from the synergism of an unknown immune mechanism plus the cytoxic effect of drugs upon tumor cells.

We have attempted to reveal this synergism in another experimental system. The WO strain of human uterine choriocarcinoma was transplanted into the cheek pouches of four groups of cortison-

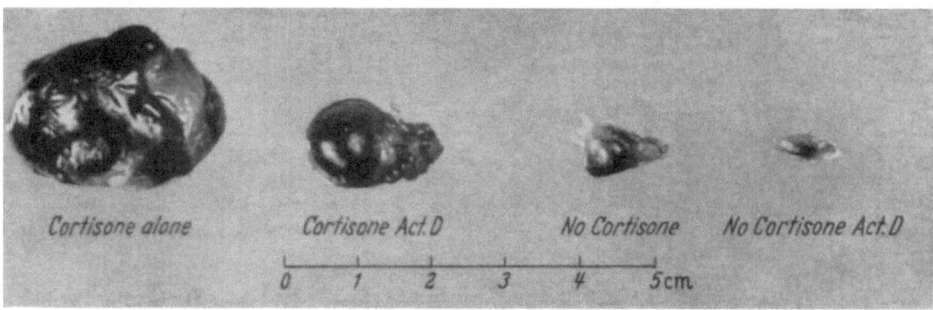

Fig. 5. Synergism of immunity and drug effect

or not there is a transplantation immunity, we have attempted to demonstrate this serologically. The tanned red cell agglutination technique with choriocarcinoma protein serving as an antigen, was used. Our results, based on the sera of ten patients, have failed to reveal any significantly high titre of anti-tumor antibody regardless of the status of disease of the patients, whether in complete remission or in progressive dissemination. Contrary to these findings, are the data recently reported by Mathe et al., (1964), who found that the sera of three of six women with trophoblastic disease agglutinnated their husbands' white blood corpuscles. Whether or not this is an unrelated phenomenon due to sensitization from previous normal pregnancies, has to be further evaluated.

ized hamsters. In Group a, the hamsters continued to receive cortisone twice weekly throughout the entire experimental period to suppress heterograft rejection. In Group b, the hamsters received cortisone similarly, but on the seventh day after the transplant, when the tumors were in maximum growth rate, Actinomycin D, 5 micrograms, was given intraperitoneally each day for five consecutive days. In Group c, maintenance cortisone was withdrawn from the seventh day after transplant to allow tumor rejection to occur. In Group d, maintenance cortisone was withdrawn similar to Group c, but in addition, the hamsters received Actinomycin D identical to those in Group b.

One will note from Figure 5, that the smallest average tumor size was in Group d, showing the synergism of drug effect and transplantation immunity. Tumor size of Groups b and c was substantially smaller than that of Group a which received cortisone maintenance and was without drug therapy.

Our experience with 28 patients with advanced uterine trophoblastic tumor confirms the findings that teratogenic drugs such as methotrexate, actinomycin D, 6-diazo-5-oxo-L-norleucine, and alkylating agents cause tumor regression. Some of the tumor regressions are complete and have been sustained for a long duration, from five to eight years. On the other hand, testicular choriocarcinoma has not responded regularly and satisfactorily to the above drugs when given separately. Nevertheless, combination of the three classes of drugs, namely, Chlorambucil, Methotrexate and Actinomycin D, induce complete or partial tumor regression in 50% of the subjects with

testicular choriocarcinoma. The average duration of response is six moths. Rarely, complete tumor regression can be sustained more than two years.

The reason for the difference in therapeutic response, is partly attributed to the difference in tumor sensitivity to the drugs used, and partly to the difference in host-tumor relationship. Metastatic uterine choriocarcinoma is essentially a homologous transplant to the host, thus theoretically subject to immunological rejection. Metastatic testicular choriocarcinoma is an auto-transplant, and no immunological rejection is expected. Although we have failed to demonstrate transplantation immunity in women with uterine trophoblastic tumors, our other experimental data can be interpreted to suggest that synergism of an immune mechanism and drug therapy is contributing to the success of obtaining long-term tumor regression.

References

BROWN, J. H., and KENNEDY, B. J., Mithramycin in the treatment of disseminated testicular neoplasms. *New Engl. J. Med.* **272**, 111—118 (1965).

GRACE J. T., Jr. Discussion of the paper entitled "Induced immunity to cancer cell homografts in man", by SOUTHAM, C. M., and MOORE, A. E. *Am. N. Y. Acid. Sci.* **73**, 651-653 (1958).

LI, M. C., HERTZ, R. and BERGENSTAL, D. M., Therapy of choriocarcinoma and related trophoblastic tumors with folic acid and purine antagonists. *New Engl. J. Med.* **259**, 66-74 (1958).

— WHITMORE, W. F., Jr., GOLDBERG, R., and GRABSTALD, H., Effects of combined drug

therapy on metastatic cancer of testis. *J. Amer. med Ass.* **174**, 1291-1299).

MACKENZIE, A. R., Personal communication, speech given to the New York Cancer Society in December 1964.

MATHE, G., DAUSSET, J., HERRET, E., AMIEL, J. L., COLOMBANI, J., and BRULE, G., Immunological studies in patients with placental choriocarcinoma. *J. nat. Cancer Inst.* **33**, 193-208 (1964).

ROBINSON, E., SHULMAN, J., BEN-HUR, N., ZUCKERMAN, H., and NEUMAN, Z., Immunological studies and behavior of husband and foreign homografts in patients with chorioepithelioma. *Lancet*, **1963** I, 300—302.

Synopsis of discussion V

Dr. HSU presented the clinical and autopsy findings of a 43 year old multipara who developed choriocarcinoma following a curettage for threatened abortion. During methotrexate treatment she manifested signs of central nerv-

ous system metastasis and despite continuous vigorous application of the drug, died. During the course of her treatment, cutaneous and mucosal metastates had sloughed out. At autopsy brain metastases were surrounded by plasma cells, lymphocytes, and polymorphonuclear leukocytes. These findings were interpreted to implicate immunologic participation in tumor rejection in this patient.

Dr. BILLINGHAM remarked that on the whole, evidence presented throughout the Conference tended to make the case for an immunological factor, in part responsible for regression of trophoblastic neoplasia in women, less credible as more evidence was available. He cited Dr. LI's important evidence that in no case of histologically regressing tumor material he had seen was there evidence of mononuclear cell infiltration. This made him reluctant to entertain seriously the idea that any form of weak homograft resistance was playing a part in the drug-facilitated regression of these tumors. Dr. HSU's case was considered a rare exception. A possibility that remains open is that organ or tissue specific antigens are involved, not an isoantigen which is genetically determined. If this be the case, one might be able to examine such a hypothesis by serum transfers from patients with prior regressions to patients with active disease. It should put the concept of immunologic resistance to test.

If one still believes there is synergistic effect between drugs and actively acquired immunity, an experimental approach worthy of examination would involve mice previously mated with males of another strain. If pre-existing specific sensitization against the transplantation antigens of these males, possibly induced by skin homografting were present, it might be effective in terminating pregnancy in association with methotrexate at dose levels which methotrexate could not accomplish alone. This thus would test the hypothesis that normal trophoblast is weakly isoantigenetic. Dr. BILLINGHAM admitted a great onus on biologists working on transplantation immunology

to attempt once and for all to determine whether the normal trophoblast does contain transplantation antigens. As a step toward this knowledge he advocated that appropriate investigators study the fate of chorionepithelioma transplanted into human volunteers.

Dr. BILLINGHAM cautioned that in interpreting tolerance to homografts from the husband, one should consider data derived in mice that repeated pregnancy in one strain by a male mouse of another strain may lead to a specific immunologic tolerance to transplantation of the father's strain. Thus some of the apparent tolerance of the husband's skin grafting may relate to multiparity. Dr. BILLINGHAM interpreted the occurrence of successful pregnancy after chemotherapeutic cure as a telling argument against the participation of acquired immunologic activity in the prior regression. An even more conclusive point of evidence would be spontaneous cure followed by a normal pregnancy. Such an event, he believed, would ring the death knell of the immunologic hypothesis. Dr. BREWER remarked that the spontaneous regression of choriocarcinoma is not at all common. There is but a single instance among 270 choriocarcinomas in the Mathieu Registry. Dr. ACOSTA-SISON agreed that she had never seen a spontaneous regression of choriocarcinoma. There was concensus however, that spontaneous regression of metastatic mole occurs not infrequently.

Dr. HERTZ clarified his view on the dissimilarity in therapeutic response of testicular choriocarcinoma and gestational trophoblastic neoplasms of women. He pointed out that the comparable tumor in the female was the nongestational gonadal trophoblastic neoplasm and his experience with this tumor and testicular choriocarcinoma had been uniformly unfavorable. Both are autochthonous tumors. The choriocarcinomatous element of the neoplasms respond brilliantly to the drugs described with dramatic drop in gonadotropin hormone excretion. When the choriocarcinomatous element becomes resistant to drug, however, or where it initially was present as one of several tissue constituents of the tumor, as usually is the case, the outcome is unfavorable, since the other neoplastic elements in the testicular or ovarian tumors are quite resistant to the drugs now available.

Dr. Li reported that men with teratocarcinoma, embryonal carcinoma, or choriocarcinoma respond equally well to combination chemotherapy, although the responses are usually transient. In one instance a man with teratocarcinoma and embryonal carcinoma has been in complete remission for five years following chemotherapy for multiple pulmonary metastases.

Integration of Treatment Methods
in Trophoblastic Growths

Myroslaw M. Hreshchyshyn, M. D., and James F. Holland, M. D.

*State University of New York Medical School at Buffalo
and Roswell Park Memorial Institute, Buffalo, N. Y.*

Our concepts of abnormal trophoblastic growth and its management are changing under the influence of advances made with chemotherapy. We must compare each newly advocated principle with the old, however, and make it prove its superiority. We should not discard accumulated knowledge before the era of chemotherapy simply because it is old, and simply because new alternatives exist.

The curative value of chemotherapy in treatment of patients with trophoblatic growth is an established fact. Chemotherapy, however, is not without hazards, may be unnecessary in some cases, and does not cure all patients with trophoblastic growth. Furthermore, there are patients who fail on chemotherapy who may still be cured with surgery. Prevention and one hundred per cent curability of abnormal trophoblastic growth with chemotherapy remain the objective of our research, but until this is achieved it will be necessary to integrate the available methods of chemotherapy with the overall management of these diseases.

Before considering therapy, it is necessary to reach a consensus about the various forms of trophoblastic growths and their malignity. The classification in Appendix I, proposed to this conference by the Committee on Nomenclature, serves well for this purpose.

The degree of clinical malignity of the growth does not always correlate with its morphology. Perhaps it is a function of the relationship between the host and the tumor. Consequently the choice of treatment in an individual case is not determined solely by the growth's morphology but more by the clinical behavior of the tumor and the extent of tumor spread. It must be conceded, however, that as a group, patients with invasive and metastatic hydatidiform mole have a much better prognosis than patients with choriocarcinoma (Hreshchyshyn et al. 1961).

Securing a histologic diagnosis is of importance for future evaluation of any treatment method and should be sought in every case, though not at the expense of rendering patients sterile by hysterectomy. The morphologic changes are not static in each case. In the face of persistent or recrudescent tumor, repeated biopsies where possible, would contribute greatly to our knowledge. Lumping together all forms of trophoblastic growth without critical review of the results in each is as potentially misleading, as would be considering squamous dysplasia, carcinoma in situ, and invasive carcinoma of the cervix as one entity therapeutically, even though they represent a continuum of pathologic abnormality. Clear pathologic delineation will help in evaluation of the efficiency of our treatment methods and may avoid discrepancies in cure rates achieved with chemotherapy at different clinics, otherwise explicable by admixture of varying proportions of more and less malignant diseases.

In the United States, unlike some coutries of Asia, Africa, and Latin America hydatidiform mole is relatively infrequent. There is, however, some evidence to suggest that the incidence of hydatidiform mole in the U. S. A., as in the Orient (CHUN *et al.*, 1964; PRAWIROHARDJO *et al.*, 1959), may be increasing. Review of the records from four University-affiliated general hospitals with unselected patient material from the Buffalo, New York area for the years 1954—63 revealed an increase from 1:5119 pregnancies during the first five year period to 1:2172 during the second five year period. For the corresponding periods of time the incidence of hydatidiform mole among patients who aborted increased from 1:435 to 1:233. If this trend continues an increase in the incidence of choriocarcinoma may also be anticipated.

Hydatidiform mole, non-invasive, is treated simply be evacuating it from the uterine cavity. To prevent the development of invasive hydatidiform mole, of metastatic growth, and of choriocarcinoma prophylactic regimens have been advocated. Liberal performance of hysterectomy as a primary treatment (ACOSTA-SISON, 1964), routine recurettage of the uterus one week following evacuation of the mole (COPPLESON, 1958) and prophylactic chemotherapy all have been suggested. Hysterectomy may be a justifiable procedure in selected patients where

childbearing is no longer desired. Because of the relative infrequency of malignant transformation of hydatidiform mole and because the subsequent development of malignant trophoblastic growth is not necessarily prevented by primary hysterectomy, wide acceptance of this procedure cannot be advised.

The value of routine recurettage and of prophylactic chemotherapy could only be determined in well controlled studies by a group of clinics with access to a large number of patients. The reported results with the use of amethopterin in small series of patients with hydatidiform mole in the prophylaxis of malignant growths are quite encouraging and justify further studies. For the present, however, close follow-up of all patients who had hydatidiform mole with reliance on clinical signs and accurate chorionic gonadotropin titers remains the standard procedure. If four or six weeks after evacuation of the mole the uterus remains subinvoluted, there is metrorrhagia, or if there is persistent elevation of gonadotropin the uterine cavity should be curetted for remnants of hydatidiform mole. If at curettage molar tissue is removed but the uterus subsequently does not involute or the titer disappear, a third curettage is indicated. Removal of the remaining mole is usually followed by uterine involution and decrease of gonadotropin titer to a normal level. The patient then should be examined and the gonadotropin titer determined frequently at first and at progressively longer intervals for at least a year so as to detect any recrudescence that might occur.

Patients with persistently elevated gonadotropin levels despite negative curettage are suspect of harboring hydatidiform mole outside the uterine cavity. Our philosophy of managing such patients is reflected in Table I. First, it is important to establish whether the gona-

Table I. *Management of hydatidiform mole with "pregnancy test" positive 4—6 weeks after curettage, Buffalo, 1958—64*

Treatment	No.	Metastases None	Vagina	Lung	Unknown site	Titer Unchanged or rising	Decreased	Alive-No disease	Survival years
Hysterectomy	1[1]	1				1		1	2
VCR + Hysterectomy	1[1]			1		1		1	3
MTX	4			3	1[2]	4		4	6, 4, 4, 1
Di. Cl. Mtx		5	1[3]						
No Treatment	6						6	6	4, 4, 3, 1, 1, 1/2
Total	12	6	1	4	1	6	6	12	

[1] Elderly multipara. — [2] Had prior hysterectomy for invasive mole; persistent elevation of H.C.G. — [3] Vaginal metastases diagnosed and excised prior to Dx and evacuation of mole. VCR = Vincristine. MTX = Methotrexate. Di. Cl. Mtx = Dichloromethotrexate.

dotropin titer is falling or rising. Two determinations should be done one week apart. If it is falling the patient should be followed at two week intervals with pelvic examination and gonadotropin titer determinations. Spontaneous regression of metastatic mole is well known and if the titer continues to fall, observation alone is indicated. For an older multiparous patient without detectable metastases, hysterectomy is still the procedure of choice. It has been suggested that surgery may lead to dissemination of the mole and thereby to pulmonary metastases (COCKSHOTT, 1964; HENDRICKSE, personal communication). There is need for further study of this. If established, some form of chemotherapy then would supercede surgery even for the elderly multipara. If pulmonary metastases do appear after curettage or hysterectomy chemotherapy should be instituted. All young patients in whom it is desired to preserve childbearing capacity, and old patients who after hysterectomy have persistent elevation of gonadotropin should be treated with chemotherapy. Suitable baseline clinical, radiologic and hormone parameters must be established. A more aggressive attitude may be required in some patients with rapid progression of tumor growth and in clinics where adequate follow-up is not possible.

The question of the relative value of hysterectomy versus chemotherapy in patients with choriocarcinoma confined to the uterus is difficult to settle because of the often inconclusive nature of diagnosis from curettings alone. Where childbearing is a factor, chemotherapy should be used before hysterectomy. There is no evidence that hysterectomy has any value in patients with disseminated choriocarcinoma (HRESHCHYSHYN et al., 1961).

Our own experience with chemotherapy in women with frank disseminated histologically confirmed choriocarcinoma is shown in Table II. Eight were of gestational and one of teratomatous origin. Two out of eight patients treated with methotrexate responded by complete disappearance of the tumors for eight and seven years respectively. One patient who failed on methotrexate responded to dichloromethotrexate and another to actinomycin D and they are alive and free of detectable disease five years and one year later. A 60 year old patient with non-gestational choriocarcinoma of teratomatous origin who was effectively palliated with vincristine deserves special mention (Picture 1). Later when her disease reactivated she was treated with methotrexate but failed to respond.

the original report by LI, HERTZ, and SPENCER (1956) and subsequent extensive and favorable experience with this drug by HERTZ and others (1961) and as further extended in this monograph by HERTZ.

Favorable results in the treatment of malignant trophoblastic growth with 6-mercaptopurine have been reported by SUNG and others of Peking (1964). In the experience of BAGSHAWE from London (1963), and HENDRICKSE from Ibadan, Nigeria (personal communication), the

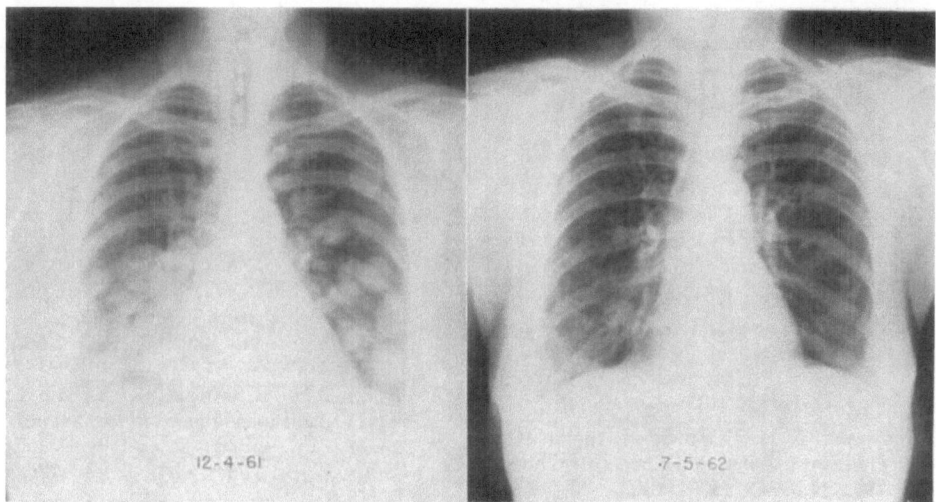

Picture 1

Table II. *Disseminated choriocarcinoma in women in Buffalo, 1956—63*

Drugs	Primary chemotherapy			Secondary chemotherapy			Alive	Years duration
	No.	C.R.	P.R.	No.	C.R.	P.R.		
Mtx	7	2	2	1*	0	0	2	8,7
Di. Cl. Mtx	1	—	—	1	1	—	1	5
Act D	—	—	—	1	1	—	1	1
VCR	1*	—	1	—	—	—	—	—
TSPA	—	—	—	2	—	—	—	—
Total	9	2	3	1	2	—	4	

* A 60 year-old patient with choriocarcinoma of teratomatous origin.

Mtx = Methotrexate. Di. Cl. Mtx = Dichloromethotrexate. Act D = Actinomycin D. VCR = Vincristine. TSPA = Triethylenethiophosphoramide. No. = Number, C. R. = Complete remission. P. R. = Partial remission.

In the United States, methotrexate is the drug of choice when chemotherapy in indicated. This is largely because of

combination of methotrexate and 6-MP gave better results than might have been expected from either drug alone.

Where therapy including methotrexate fails, other drugs, e. g. actinomycin D, vinblastine, and DON may still produce a cure. DON, according to KARNOFSKY (this conference), is not likely to be effective in patients who failed to respond to Amethopterin and actinomycin D (1964). When these drugs fail, others, e. g. nitromin, chlorambucil, mitomycin C. dichloromethotrexate, vincristine, podophylline derivatives (STOMM 1964) and also ionizing radiation may be considered in patients with disseminated growth. AINBINDER et al. from Leningrad (1946), recently reported good results with the use of antibiotic 2703 (chryso-malin. Surgery should be employed when growth is resectable. Hysterectomy or hysterotomy should be done when the tumor is confined to the uterus. Angiography may be helpful in localizing the tumor (COCKSHOTT et al., 1964). Patients with distant regionalized metastases can sometimes be cured by excision of the tumor (HRESHCHYSHYN et al., 1961).

In summary, we would like to stress the need for integration of available treatment methods, discrimination with regard to clinical malignity of the growth, and comparative evelution based on a uniform and meaningful classification of trophoblastic neoplasia.

References

ACOSTA-SISON, H., Changing attitudes in the management of hydatidiform mole. Amer. J. Obstet. Gynec. 88, 634—636 (1964).

AINBINDER, N. M., DILMAN, V. M., MUKHINA, E. P., NECHAEVA, I. D., and SHARKOVA, J. M., The use of the antibiotic 2703 in six cases of chorioepethelioma of the uterus. Vop. Onkol. 10, 103—107 (1964).

BAGSHAWE, K. D., Trophoblastic tumors. Chemotherapy and developments. Brit. med. J. 1963, No 5368, 1303—1307.

COPPLESON, M., Hydatidiform mole and its complications. J. Obstet. Gynaec. Brit. Emp. 65, 238—252 (1958).

CHUN, D., BRAGA, C., CHOW, C., and LOK, L., Clinical observations on some aspects of hydatidiform moles. J. Obstet. Gynaec. Cwlth. 71, 180—184 (1964).

COCKSHOTT, W. P., EVANS, K. T., and HENDRICKSE, J. P., Arteriography of trophoblastic tumors. Clin Radiol. 15, 1—8 (1964).

HENDRICKSE, J. P.: Personal communication.

HERTZ, R., LEWIS, J., Jr., and LIPSETT, M. B.: Five years' experience with the chemotherapy of metastatic choriocarinoma and related trophoblastic tumors in women. Am. J. Obst. Gynec. 82, 631—640 (1961).

HRESHCHYSHYN, M. M., GRAHAM, J. B., and HOLLAND J. F., Treatment of malignant trophoblastic growth in women, with special reference to amethopterin. Amer. J. Obstet. Gynec. 81, 688—705 (1961).

KARNOFSKY, D. A., GOLBEY, R. B., and LI, M. C., Remissions induced in trophoblastic tumors by 6-diazo-5-oxo-L-Norleucine (DON). Proc. Amer. Ass. Cancer Res. 5, 33 (1964).

LI, M. C., HERTZ, R., and SPENCER, D. B., Effect of methotrexate therapy upon choriocarcinoma and chorioadenoma. Proc. Soc. exp. Biol. (N. Y.) 93, 361—366 (1956).

PRAWIROHARDJO, S. et al: Hydatidiform mole and choriocarcinoma in Indonesia. Ist Asiatic Obstet. Gynec. (Tokyo) 1959, p. 112.

STAMM, O., Cancer therapy with podophyllin derivates. Münch. med. Wschr. 106, 41—48 (1964).

SUNG, H., WU, P. C., and HO, T. H., Treatment of choriocarcinoma and chorioadenoma destruens with 6-MP and surgery. Acta Un. int. contra Cancr. 20, 493—502 (1964).

Synopsis of discussion VI

The report of the morphology committee under the chairmanship of Dr. ISHIZUKA, including Drs. PARK, BREWER, HERTZ, and HRESHCHYSHYN was accepted. It is published as Appendix I. Syncytial endometritis is excluded as a type of neoplastic trophoblastic phenomenon, since it represents a histologic entity of the endometrium responding to trophoblastic neoplasia which may be occult elsewhere. Thus, patients with a histologic diagnosis of syncytial endometritis who die from choriocarcinoma do not succumb to metastases from the syncytial endometritis but from the trophoblastic neoplasia not found at the time of curettage. Furthermore, syncytial endometritis may be found in normal pregnancies and in the post-partum period either after abortion or term gestation.

Dr. HOLLAND remarked that it had become clear at the Conference that a drug is not a drug per se, but only when discussed in terms of its dose, the duration of its administration, and the route and schedule by which it is administered. It is necessary to be cautious concerning the evaluation of particular therapies since inadequate dose or inappropriate administration might compromise the results obtained. He believed that a comparative study carried out concomitantly would have made many of the data available more interpretable. Despite all the ancillary techniques of objective measurement, a body of clinical data using a uniform technique of therapy is not as interpretable as data from a critically controlled comparative study. Modifications in professional staff, changes in ancillary therapy such as transfusions, antibiotics and surgery, compromise the ability to compare a uniform therapeutic experience with some prior experience. He advocated designed planned programs of study in which one new therapeutic step at a time was undertaken to attain proof of therapeutic superiority rather than clinical impression.

Dr. HOLLAND stressed that since recrudesence of the disease occurred early after therapeutic failure in most instances it was unnecessary to talk in terms of five

year survivals, but rather in terms of cure. Dr. HERTZ has a patient with $8\,^1/_2$ years of survival. Dr. HOLLAND has a patient with 8 years of survival and there are many others shorter who have not relapsed. Thus discussions in terms of cure are appropriate. Methotrexate and actinomycin D clearly seemed capable of curative activity. Mithramycin, an antibiotic with reported activity in non-gestational gonadotropin secreting neoplasms of the testis might be considered for study in gestational trophoblastic neoplasia of women.

Dr. HOLLAND advocated consideration of disease in terms of the actual occurrences to the patient, rather than arbitrary time. Tumor size, extent of tumor metastasis, evidences of impact on the host, and similar parameters might account for the actual influence which is expressed in time. He advocated a substantial effort to determine whether prophylactic chemotherapy is valid. Studies should be conducted with adequate controls so that proof of the hypothesis might be obtained rather than a body of experience which might have to be compared to another experience in a separate clinic by a different individual. He stressed the beauty of gonadotropin assay by techniques which eliminate animal testing because of the inherently greater reproducibility and potentially greater sensitivity.

Dr. BURCHENAL outlined studies for the future. He stressed the merit of discovering the reason for excellent response in trophoblastic neoplasia to methotrexate treatment. He questioned whether exquisite sensitivity to each of the drugs was the critical phenomenon or whether a question of host defense was pertinent. He reiterated the importance of dose scheduling in treatment with methotrexate or with diaza-oxo-L-norleucine (DON) where spaced dosing was less toxic than when the drug was given daily or more often. Similar information is available for mouse neoplasms with cyclophosphamide treatment. He thought that suitable experimental systems might be the choriocarcinomas carried in hamster cheek pouch by Dr. HERTZ, or possibly transplanted mouse leukemias. All the agents which have worked in choriocarcinoma to date are also active in mouse leukemia.

Dr. BURCHENAL thought that in the instances where chemotherapeutic resistance occurs in trophoblastic neoplasia, new drugs might be best used. Another possibility is the combined application of 6-mercaptopurine and DON. Nearly 10 years previously, he had shown that this combination was exceptionally good in mouse leukemia and with it he was unable to develop a resistant line. With either mercaptopurine or DON alone, resistance occurs fairly rapidly in mouse leukemia and has been recognized for each in choriocarcinoma. In patients with leukemia, there did not seem to be any prevention of the emergence of resistance when 6-mercaptopurine and DON were used simultaneously. Since both agents independently are active in choriocarcinoma, however, considerably improved results might be anticipated.

Dr. BURCHENAL also thought that fluorouracil or fluorodeoxyuridine might well be tried, as well as cytosine arabinoside. Vincristine is more active in acute leukemia in children then vinblastine and despite its additional neurotoxicity might be a valuable agent for use in choriocarcinoma. The terephthalanilides are of great experimental interest and are active in mouse leukemia. They might eventually find a place in treatment of choriocarcinoma.

Dr. HOLLAND indicated the desirability not only of translating information from mouse tumor screens to human disease, but from efficacy in one human disease to another. He emphasized the therapeutic superiority of methotrexate given twice weekly in remission to children with acute lymphocytic leukemia and advanced it as a candidate treatment regimen in trophoblastic neoplasia.

Dr. HERTZ stressed the need to delineate criteria for the evaluation of response. This has been necessitated by a revision of concepts on the relation of various phases of trophoblastic neoplasia one to another. He also expressed the opinion that trial of new drugs in resistant patients would be at considerable handicap. As time elapsed during the trophoblastic residence in the maternal host, he believed there was progressive loss of the potential for complete remission. Thus a new agent might be tried in a biological system inherently less responsive than that disease earlier treated by the more standard agents. He believed effective evaluation of new agents might of necessity require new cases. The clinical and ethical considerations to undertake this are indeed complex. He thought the only realistic recourse was the use of animal experimental systems by analogy. The choriocarcinoma system in the hamster is subject to definite discrepancies from effects which might be expected in man. The development of resistance in the tumor in the hamster is quite different from the tumor when it was in the patient. Accordingly, there must be substantial reservation in accepting the screening data directly with respect to their potential clinical value.

Dr. HERTZ emphasized the need for accuracy and precision in gonadotropic hormone assay and he hoped that immunoassay or radioimmunoassay would permit some of the difficulties in this area to be overcome. He believed evaluation of gonadotropin excretion was the key to successful chemotherapy of choriocarcinoma, because of the sensitivity and reliability provided by the hormone assay and its relationship to the presence of tumor.

Dr. HRESHCHYSHYN stressed the desirability of accurate differentiation between hydatidiform mole and pregnancy. Possibly increased reliability of and technicologic advances in estrogen determination might make this distinction easier. Dr. HRESHCHYSHYN acknowledged the usefulness of animal tumor screens. He postulated that if new drugs could be tested on normal trophoblast, additional information would be available. This has always been difficult because chemotherapy affected the embryo, and after embryonic death, uterine expulsion or absorption of the placenta occurred. He has employed methotrexate in one patient with abdominal pregnancy where the placenta had been left behind and observed methotrexate effect on normal trophoblast. He has worked experimentally attempting to grow normal placenta in extrauterine sites in normal animals.

Dr. PAI expressed hope that a combined clinical trial be established in which help could be given to women in the underdeveloped countries. He acknowledged a handicap in the conduct of bioassays, in the critical pathological evaluation of specimens, and in drug supply. Abundant clinical material and patients in need however, provided solid basis for joining East and West together. He recounted trials in tuberculosis and the treatment of smallpox and hoped that a similar venture in choriocarcinoma could be projected.

Dr. KOBAYASHI expressed interest in seeing an international registry of trophoblastic neoplasia established much as the international registry for cancer of the cervix.

Dr. KOSS stressed the provocative observation that anticancer drugs can produce cancer-like changes in benign tissues recognizable cytologically. It should have significant bearing on future studies because as patients are cured of one neoplasm by chemotherapeutic means the possible carcinogenic activity of the agents used, may, many years later, elicit other cancers. He thus urged close attention to second neoplasms developing in patients successfully treated chemotherapeutically for choriocarcinoma who had survived for many years.

Dr. NELSON expressed admiration for Dr. ISHIZUKA's observations that the return of normal ovulatory cycles may put patients in a safe category following hydatidiform mole. Those whose ovulatory cycles do not return may be the ones most in need of prophylactic therapy and this may be a simple way of predicting the troublesome patient for the future, and thus a way select the group at greatest risk. Dr. ISHIZUKA added that one patient who had ovulatory cycles did proceed to the development of neoplasm.

Dr. BORJA expressed pride that the Philippines was the host country for the Conference, and closed the proceedings.

Appendix I

Trophoblastic Neoplasia

A. Gestational.

B. Non-gestational.

I. CLINICAL DIAGNOSIS.

1. Non-metastatic.
2. Metastatic.
   a. Local (pelvic).
   b. Extra-pelvic (specify location).
3. Other required information.
   a. Evidence.
      i. Morphologic.
      ii. Non-morphologic.
   b. Antecedent pregnancy. Specify duration.
      i.   Normal.
      ii. Abortal.
      iii. Molar.
   c. Previous treatment.
      i. Untreated.
      ii. Treated. Specify.

II. MORPHOLOGIC DIAGNOSIS.

1. Hydatidiform mole.
   a. Non-invasive.
   b. Invasive.
2. Choriocarcinoma.
3. Uncertain[1].
4. Other required information.
   a. Diagnostic basis. Specify.
      i.   C = Curettage.
      ii. U = Excised uterus.
      iii. N = Necropsy.
      iv. O = Other.
   b. Date of diagnosis (with respect to date of onset of treatment.
   c. Subsequent change in morphologic diagnosis. Specify diagnostic basis as in II. 4a.

---

[1] "Syncytial endometritis" *not* considered neoplasia.

Appendix II

Choriocarcinoma conference lecture award citation to
ROY HERTZ, M. D., Ph. D.

For Distinguished Service to Mankind

(Delivered by JAMES F. HOLLAND, M. D.)

You were an author of the first paper reporting the use of a folic antagonist chemotherapeutic treatment for cancer which has proved curative. You persevered in this work. You concentrated your own talents on trophoblastic tumors and effectively deployed the skills and resources of others. After MIN CHIU LI, your co-discoverer, moved to another hospital, you trained and led other physicians and scientists. You mobilized the enormous resources of your institution to meld an unequalled organization for the study and treatment of tumors of the chorion.

You have firmly established by extended experience and unremitting effort that the initial observations were true. You have introduced other chemotherapeutic treatments that can cure chorionic tumors if the initial treatment fails.

You have published your results with clarity and dispatch so that other members of the world scientific and medical community could learn from your teachings, and having learned, could also cure cancer chemotherapeutically.

From the perspective of only 10 years, one might cavil that this is a special tumor and a special circumstance. With an eye toward the stark beauty of truth yet to come, however, such is a blurry view. This will be one of the great landmarks of cancer research, and other cures of other cancers must surely follow, building in part on the lessons learned in the past decade.

As cancer research moves to new challenges and new successes in the next decade we can confidently predict that you will be in the vanguard. This Choriocarcinoma Conference Lecture Award is thus presented to you, ROY HERTZ, in recognition and appreciation of your distinguished service to mankind through cancer research.

UICC Publications

Kaposi's Sarcoma. S. Karger AG., Basle (Switzerland) — New York (1963).

Cancer of the urinary bladder. S. Karger AG., Basle (Switzerland) — New York (1963).

Prognosis of malignant tumours of the breast. S. Karger AG., Basle (Switzerland) — New York (1963).

The lymphoreticular tumours in Africa. S. Karger AG., Basle (Switzerland) — New York (1964).

Cellular control mechanisms and cancer. Elsevier Publishing Company, Amsterdam — London — New York (1964).

Illustrated Tumor Nomenclature. Springer-Verlag, Berlin — Heidelberg — New York (1965).